T0201791

# Human Oral Mucosa

## Development, Structure, and Function

# Human Oral Mucosa

## Development, Structure, and Function

Edited by

Christopher Squier, PhD, DSc,
FRCPath (Lond)
Kim A. Brogden, PhD

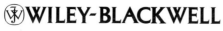

A John Wiley & Sons, Inc., Publication

# Contents

# Preface

It is almost 35 years since the first edition of *Human Oral Mucosa: Development, Structure, and Function* was published by Blackwell Scientific Publications. When this volume originally appeared, the intent was to provide a more comprehensive account of the oral mucosa than was available in textbooks of histology and dental anatomy at the time. Reviews of the volume were favorable, and it was evident that it met the needs not only of dental students but also of dental practitioners and academic pathologists and dermatologists.

One of the reasons, therefore, for proposing the present volume was to provide a more sophisticated text on oral mucosa than presently exists in textbooks or in any separate, specialist volume. In the absence of alternate texts, it seemed appropriate to update the original text to reflect the considerable increase in our knowledge of oral mucosa that has occurred in recent years. Our understanding of the structure of oral mucosa is now established at a molecular rather than a tissue or cellular level. This in turn has revealed a level of function that was previously not suspected, including, for example, a sophisticated barrier to the penetration of exogenous materials, and the synthesis of specific antimicrobial compounds, representing components of the innate immune system. There is also a growing realization of commonality in structure and function between stratified squamous mucosae such as those of oral mucosa, the esophagus, and the vagina.

The new edition of *Human Oral Mucosa*, like its predecessor, is directed principally to graduate students and residents in the oral health sciences, although it will be of value to specialists in allied areas such as dermatology, internal medicine, gynecology, and pathology. In the absence of other specialist volumes in this area, we believe that it will also serve as a reference for researchers working in oral science, particularly those interested in oral infections, inflammation, HIV pathogenesis, and oral immunization.

To revise a work after such a lengthy interval reflects the encouragement and enthusiasm of our publisher and, in particular, Sophia Joyce of Wiley-Blackwell. Locally, we have had generous support from our institution and valuable input from colleagues, particularly Philip Wertz, and Catherine Davis, of Proctor and Gamble, who carefully reviewed the final chapter. Finally, we acknowledge the meticulous work of Mary Mantz who cheerfully organized the numerous figures and references for the new edition.

Christopher Squier
Kim Brogden

# Human Oral Mucosa

## Development, Structure, and Function

# The functions of oral mucosa

## 1.1 ORAL MUCOSA: WHAT IS IT AND WHAT DOES IT DO?

Oral mucosa is a *mucous membrane*, a term used to describe the moist linings of body cavities that communicate with the exterior. These include the oral cavity, nasal passages, pharynx, gastrointestinal tract, and urinogenital regions. In the oral cavity, this lining is called the *oral mucous membrane* or *oral mucosa*. The exterior of the body has a dry covering, the skin, which is continuous with oral mucosa at the lips. Structurally, the oral mucosa resembles the skin in some respects and is very similar to the mucous membranes of the esophagus, cervix, and vagina (which will be considered in a subsequent chapter) but is totally different from the gastrointestinal mucosa.

*Human Oral Mucosa: Development, Structure, and Function.* Edited by Christopher Squier and Kim A. Brogden.
© 2011 Christopher Squier and Kim A. Brogden. Published 2011 by John Wiley & Sons, Inc.

Despite these differences, skin and the different mucosae all consist of two structurally different tissue components: a covering epithelium and an underlying connective tissue. These tissues function together so the various mucosae and skin can be considered as organs.

Form follows function, and it is easier to understand the complex structure of a tissue or organ when its function is known. This is particularly true of the oral mucosa, whose structure reflects a variety of functional adaptations. The major adaptations are a result of evolutionary changes that have taken place over a long time. However, small and usually reversible changes in structure of oral mucosa may be seen in response to function during the lifetime of an individual, but these are not heritable. The functions of oral mucosa and the tissue components subserving those functions are summarized in Table 1.1.

**Table 1.1**  Functions of the oral mucosa.

| Function | | | Structures involved |
|---|---|---|---|
| Protection | Mechanical role | Friction/abrasion | Epithelium (stratum corneum) |
| | | Compression/shearing | Lamina propria (collagen/elastin) |
| | Barrier role | Molecules | Epithelium (superficial barrier) |
| | | Microorganisms | |
| Sensory | Taste | | Epithelium (taste buds) |
| | Touch, temperature, pain | | Epithelium and lamina propria (sensory receptors) |
| Synthesis/secretion | Saliva | | Minor salivary glands (lamina propria, submucosa) |
| | Sebum | | Sebaceous glands (lamina propria) |
| Esthetics | | | Vermilion border of lips |

# 1.2 FUNCTIONS OF THE ORAL MUCOSA

The oral mucosa has a variety of functions of which the most important is protection of the deeper tissues and glands of the oral cavity. Other functions include sensory perception, synthesis, and secretion from glands located in the mucosa and an esthetic role represented by the mucocutaneous junction.

## 1.2.1 Protection

As a surface lining, the oral mucosa separates and protects deeper tissues and organs in the oral region from the environment of the oral cavity. The normal activities of seizing, biting, and chewing food expose the oral soft tissues to mechanical forces (compression, stretching, shearing) and surface abrasions (from hard particles in the diet). The oral mucosa shows a number of adaptations of both the epithelium and the connective tissue to withstand these mechanical insults. Furthermore, there is normally a resident population of microorganisms within the oral cavity that would cause infection if they gained access to the tissues. Many of these organisms also produce substances that have a toxic effect on tissues. The epithelium of the oral mucosa acts as the major barrier to penetration and also contributes to the immunoprotective system of the mucosa.

## 1.2.2 Sensation

The sensory function of the oral mucosa is important because it provides considerable information about events within the oral cavity, whereas the lips and tongue perceive stimuli outside the mouth. In the mouth, pharynx and epiglottis are receptors that respond to temperature, touch, and pain; there also are the taste buds, which are not found anywhere else in the body. These signal the traditional taste sensations of sweet, salty, sour, bitter, and umami (or savory), although it has been suggested recently that there is a "fat" taste (Laugerette et al., 2007). Certain receptors in the oral mucosa probably respond to the "taste" of water and signal the satisfaction of thirst (de Araujo et al., 2003). Reflexes such as swallowing, gagging, retching, and salivating are also initiated by receptors in the oral mucosa.

### 1.2.3 Secretion

The major secretion associated with the oral mucosa is saliva, produced by the salivary glands, which contributes to the maintenance of a moist surface. The major salivary glands are situated distant from the mucosa, and their secretions pass through the mucosa via long ducts; however, many minor salivary glands are associated with the oral mucosa. Sebaceous glands are frequently present in the oral mucosa, and their secretions may have antimicrobial properties (see Chapter 2). Salivary glands secrete histatins, a family of low-molecular-weight histidine-rich proteins with antimicrobial activities. Oral epithelium is also capable of secreting a variety of antimicrobial factors such as defensins and cathelicidins, which participate in various aspects of innate immunity. These are described in Chapter 8.

### 1.2.4 Thermal regulation

In some animals (such as the dog), considerable body heat is dissipated through the oral mucosa by panting; for these animals, the mucosa plays a major role in the regulation of body temperature. The human oral mucosa, however, plays practically no role in regulating body temperature, and there are no obvious specializations of the blood vessels for controlling heat transfer such as arteriovenous shunts.

### 1.2.5 Esthetics

Skin color, texture, and appearance play an important role in signaling individual characteristics such as age, health, ethnicity, and so on. The oral mucosa is not normally visible except for the region where it joins the skin. Here, the vermilion zone of the lips represents a significant esthetic component, frequently enhanced with cosmetics in females.

## REFERENCES

de Araujo, I.E., Kringelbach, M.L., Rolls, E.T., and McGlone, F. (2003) Human cortical responses to water in the mouth, and the effects of thirst. J Neurophysiol 90(3):1865–1876.

Laugerette, F., Gaillard, D., Passilly-Degrace, P., Niot, I., and Besnard, P. (2007) Do we taste fat? Biochimie 89:265–269.

# The organization of oral mucosa

The oral cavity consists of two parts: an outer vestibule, bounded by the lips and cheeks, and the oral cavity proper, separated from the vestibule by the alveolus bearing the teeth and gingiva. The superior zone of the oral cavity proper is formed by the hard and soft palates, and the floor of the mouth and base of the tongue form the inferior border. Posteriorly, the oral cavity is bounded by the pillars of the fauces and the tonsils. The oral mucosa shows considerable structural variation in different regions of the oral cavity, but three main types of mucosa can be recognized, identified according to their primary function: masticatory mucosa, lining mucosa, and specialized mucosa. The anatomic location of each type is shown diagrammatically in Figure 2.1, and the types are fully described later in the chapter. Quantitatively, the larger part of the oral mucosa is represented by lining mucosa, amounting to approximately 60% of the total area, with masticatory mucosa and specialized mucosa occupying relatively smaller areas.

*Human Oral Mucosa: Development, Structure, and Function.* Edited by Christopher Squier and Kim A. Brogden.
© 2011 Christopher Squier and Kim A. Brogden. Published 2011 by John Wiley & Sons, Inc.

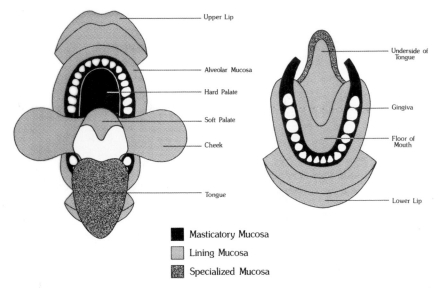

Upper Lip

Alveolar Mucosa

Hard Palate

Soft Palate

Cheek

Tongue

Underside of Tongue

Gingiva

Floor of Mouth

Lower Lip

■ Masticatory Mucosa

▢ Lining Mucosa

▨ Specialized Mucosa

**Figure 2.1** The anatomic locations of the three main types of mucosa in the oral cavity. Masticatory mucosa is shown by black shading; lining mucosa by gray shading; specialized mucosa by the stippled area. (Modified from Roed-Petersen and Renstrup, 1969, *Acta Odontol Scand* 27:681.)

## 2.1 CLINICAL FEATURES

Although the oral mucosa is continuous with the skin, it differs considerably in appearance. Generally it is more deeply colored, most obviously at the lips (where the bright vermilion zone contrasts with the skin tone). This coloration represents the combined effect of a number of factors: the concentration and state of dilation of capillaries in the underlying connective tissue, the thickness of the epithelium, the degree of keratinization, and the amount of melanin pigment in the epithelium. Color gives an indication as to the clinical condition of the mucosa; inflamed tissues are red, because of dilation of the blood vessels, whereas normal healthy tissues are a paler pink (Fig. 2.2A).

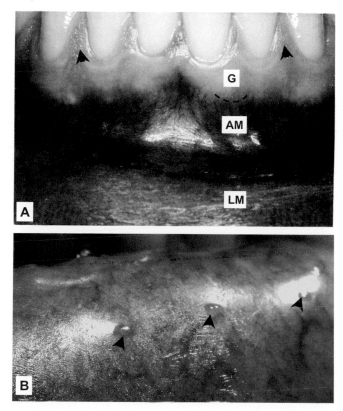

**Figure 2.2** The oral mucosa lining part of the vestibule. (A) The attached gingiva (G) is pale, and stippling is most evident in the interproximal regions (arrows). There is an abrupt junction (indicated by the dashed line) between the gingival and the alveolar mucosa (AM) which merges with the labial mucosa (LM). (B) Vermilion zone adjoining the labial mucosa. Several small globules on the mucosa *(arrows)* represent sites of secretion, where minor salivary gland ducts open to the surface.

Other features that distinguish the oral mucosa from skin are its moist surface and the absence of appendages. Skin contains numerous hair follicles, sebaceous glands, and sweat glands, whereas the glandular component of oral mucosa is represented primarily by the minor salivary glands. These are concentrated in various regions of the oral cavity, and the openings of their ducts at the mucosal surface are sometimes evident on clinical examination after drying the surface (Fig. 2.2B).

Sebaceous glands are present on the lips, labial mucosa, and buccal mucosa in over three quarters of adults and have been described occasionally in the alveolar mucosa and dorsum of the tongue. They are not associated with hair follicles and are sometimes called sebaceous follicles. Clinically, they appear as pale yellow spots (Fig. 2.3A), sometimes called *Fordyce's spots (or granules)* or *Fordyce's disease*, although they do not represent a pathologic condition.

The surface of the oral mucosa tends to be smoother and have fewer folds or wrinkles than the skin, but topographic features are readily apparent on clinical examination. The most obvious are the different papillae on the dorsum of the tongue and the transverse ridges (or rugae) of the hard palate. The healthy gingiva shows a pattern of fine surface stippling, consisting of small indentations of the mucosal

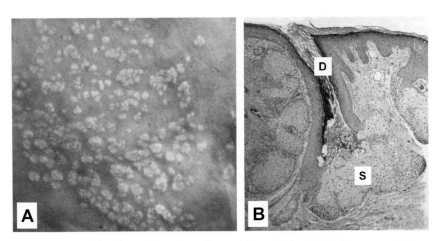

**Figure 2.3** Sebaceous glands in human buccal mucosa. (A) The "granular" appearance is clearly evident on the buccal mucosal surface. (B) Histological section of a sebaceous gland showing the secretory portion (S) and the duct (D) opening at the surface. (Photograph courtesy of Dr. M.W. Finkelstein.)

surface (Fig. 2.2A). In approximately 10% of the population, a slight whitish ridge occurs along the buccal mucosa in the occlusal plane of the teeth. This line, sometimes called the *linea alba* (white line), is a keratinized region and may represent the epithelial reaction to abrasion from rough tooth restorations or cheek biting.

The oral mucosa varies considerably in its firmness and texture. The lining mucosa of the lips and cheeks, for example, is soft and pliable, whereas the gingiva and hard palate are covered by a firm, immobile layer. These differences have important clinical implications when it comes to giving local injections of anesthetics or taking biopsies of oral mucosa. Fluid can be easily introduced into loose lining mucosa, but injection into the masticatory mucosa is more difficult and can be painful for the patient. Lining mucosa gapes when surgically incised (Fig. 2.4A) and frequently requires suturing, whereas masticatory mucosa, being more firmly attached, may not (Fig. 2.4B). Similarly, the accumulation of fluid with inflammation is obvious and painful in masticatory mucosa, but in lining mucosa the fluid disperses, and inflammation may not be so evident or as painful.

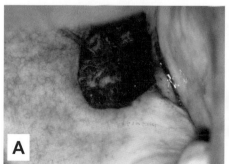
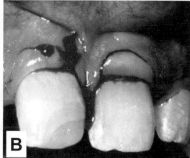

**Figure 2.4** Wounds in soft palate and gingiva. (A) A small (4 mm) biopsy wound in soft palate, a lining mucosa, results in a wound that has gaped. (B) Incisions in masticatory mucosa (attached gingiva) show little gaping of the wound. (Photograph courtesy of Dr. Georgia Johnson.)

## 2.2 COMPONENT TISSUES AND GLANDS

The two main tissue components of the oral mucosa are a stratified squamous epithelium, called the *oral epithelium*, and an underlying connective tissue layer, called the *lamina propria* (Fig. 2.5). In the skin these two tissues are known by slightly different terminology: *epidermis* and *dermis*. The interface between epithelium and connective tissue is usually irregular, and upward projections of connective tissue, called the *connective tissue papillae*, interdigitate with epithelial ridges or pegs, sometimes called the *rete ridges* or *pegs* (see Fig. 2.5). In a histological section, the interface between epithelium and connective tissue appears as a structureless

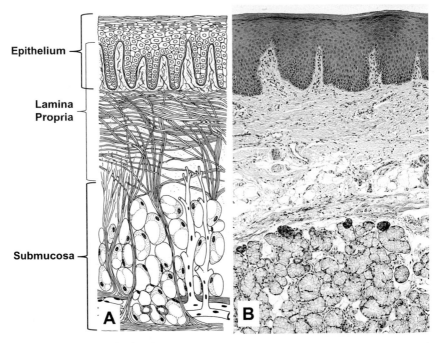

Epithelium

Lamina Propria

Submucosa

A    B

**Figure 2.5** (A) Diagram of the main tissue components of oral mucosa. (B) Histological section of hard palate to show the tissue components depicted in (A). ((A) from Squier and Finkelstein, 2003, Copyright Mosby.)

layer about 1–2 μm thick, termed the basement membrane (see Fig. 2.5B). At the ultrastructural level, this region has a complex structure (described later).

Although the junction between oral epithelium and lamina propria is obvious, that between the oral mucosa and underlying tissue, or submucosa, is less easy to recognize. In the gastrointestinal tract and esophagus, the lining mucosa is clearly separated from underlying tissues by a layer of smooth muscle and elastic fibers, the muscularis mucosae, and in functional terms may allow for some isolation of the internal lining from movements of the outer muscular layers of the intestine.

The oral mucosa has no muscularis mucosae, and clearly identifying the boundary between it and the underlying tissues is difficult. In regions such as the cheeks, lips, and parts of the hard palate, there is a layer of loose fatty or glandular connective tissue containing the major blood vessels and nerves supplying the mucosa that separates it from underlying bone or muscle. This represents the submucosa (Fig. 2.6A), and its composition determines the flexibility of the attachment of oral mucosa to the underlying structures. In regions such as the gingiva and parts of the hard palate, oral mucosa is attached directly to the periosteum of underlying bone, with no intervening submucosa

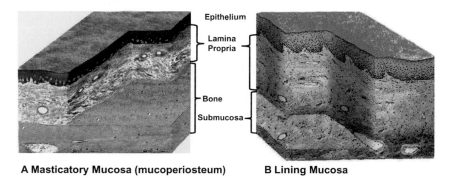

**A Masticatory Mucosa (mucoperiosteum)**　　　　**B Lining Mucosa**

**Figure 2.6** Arrangement of major tissue components in (A) masticatory mucosa (mucoperiosteum) and (B) lining mucosa.

(Fig. 2.6B). This arrangement is called a *mucoperiosteum* and provides a firm, inelastic attachment.

The minor salivary glands are situated in the submucosa of the mucosa. Sebaceous glands are less frequent than salivary glands; they lie in the lamina propria and have the same structure as those present in the skin. They produce a fatty secretion, sebum, the function of which is unclear in the oral cavity, although some claim it may lubricate the surface of the mucosa so that it slides easily against the teeth. Studies on skin suggest that sebum may have important antimicrobial properties (Drake et al., 2008), and there is some evidence for this role in oral mucosa (Wertz, P.W., personal communication).

In several regions of the oral cavity there are nodules of lymphoid tissue consisting of crypts formed by invaginations of the epithelium into the lamina propria. Capillaries in the connective tissue express adhesion molecules such as the endothelial cell leukocyte adhesion molecule (ELAM), intercellular adhesion molecule (ICAM), and vascular cell adhesion molecule (VCAM), which facilitate the trafficking of leukocytes from the blood. As a result, these areas are extensively infiltrated by lymphocytes and plasma cells. Because of their ability to mount immunologic reactions, such cells play an important role in combating infections of the oral tissues. The largest accumulations of lymphoid tissue are found in the posterior part of the oral cavity, where they form the lingual, palatine, and pharyngeal tonsils, often known collectively as *Waldeyer's ring*. Small lymphoid nodules may also sometimes occur in the mucosa of the soft palate, the ventral surface of the tongue, and the floor of the mouth.

## REFERENCES

Drake, D.R., Brogden, K.A., Dawson, D.V., and Wertz, P.W. (2008) Thematic review series: skin lipids. Antimicrobial lipids at the skin surface. J Lipid Res 49(1):4–11.

Roed-Petersen, B., and Renstrup, G. (1969) A topographical classification of the oral mucosa suitable for electronic data processing. Its application to 560 leukoplakias. Acta Odontol Scand 27:681.

Squier, C.A., and Finkelstein, M.W. (2003) Oral mucosa. In: Ten Cate's Oral Histology: Development, Structure and Function (A. Nanci, ed.) pp. 329–375. Mosby, St. Louis, MO.

# Oral epithelium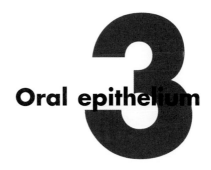

At the surface of the oral mucosa, the oral epithelium constitutes the primary barrier between the oral environment and deeper tissues. It is a stratified squamous epithelium consisting of cells tightly attached to each other and arranged in a number of distinct layers or strata. Based on the appearance in histological sections and staining with specific markers such as keratin antibodies (see section on Molecular and cellular basis of differentiation), oral epithelium can be divided into two types: keratinized epithelium, covering areas of masticatory mucosa, such as hard palate and gingiva, and non-keratinized epithelium, covering areas of lining mucosa such as cheeks, soft palate, floor of mouth. The histological appearance of these tissues is described below in more detail.

*Human Oral Mucosa: Development, Structure, and Function*. Edited by Christopher Squier and Kim A. Brogden.
© 2011 Christopher Squier and Kim A. Brogden. Published 2011 by John Wiley & Sons, Inc.

# 3.1 HISTOLOGICAL STRUCTURE OF ORAL EPITHELIUM

## 3.1.1 Keratinization

The epithelial surface of the masticatory mucosa is inflexible, tough, resistant to abrasion, and tightly bound to the lamina propria. It results from the formation of a surface layer of keratin, and the process of differentiation that produces it is called *keratinization* or *cornification*. In routine histological sections, a keratinized epithelium shows a number of distinct layers or strata (Fig. 3.1A). The basal layer (sometimes called *stratum basale*) is a layer of cuboidal or columnar cells adjacent to the basement membrane. Occasionally, the term *proliferative* or *germinative layer (stratum germinativum)* is used to describe the cells in the basal region that are capable of division, but these are functional rather than morphological terms and should be avoided in favor of basal layer. Superficial to the basal layer are several rows of larger elliptical cells known as the *prickle cell layer* or *stratum spinosum*. This term arises from the appearance of the cells prepared for histological examination; they frequently shrink away from each other, remaining in contact only at points known as intercellular bridges or desmosomes and giving the cells a spiny or prickle-like profile (Fig. 3.3A). The Greek word for prickle, *akanthe*, is often used in pathologic descriptions of an increased thickness (acanthosis) or a separation of cells caused by loss of the intercellular bridges (acantholysis) in this layer.

**Figure 3.1**   Main types of maturation in human oral epithelium. (A) Orthokeratin in ginigiva shows a narrow, darkly staining granular layer. (B) Parakeratinization in gingiva shows keratin squames that have retained pyknotic nuclei and a granular layer that contains only a few scattered granules. (C) Non-keratinization in buccal mucosa shows no clear distinction between cell strata, and nuclei are apparent in the surface layers. Note the difference in thickness and epithelial ridge pattern in addition to the patterns of maturation. ((A) and (C) from Squier and Finkelstein, 2003, Copyright Mosby.)

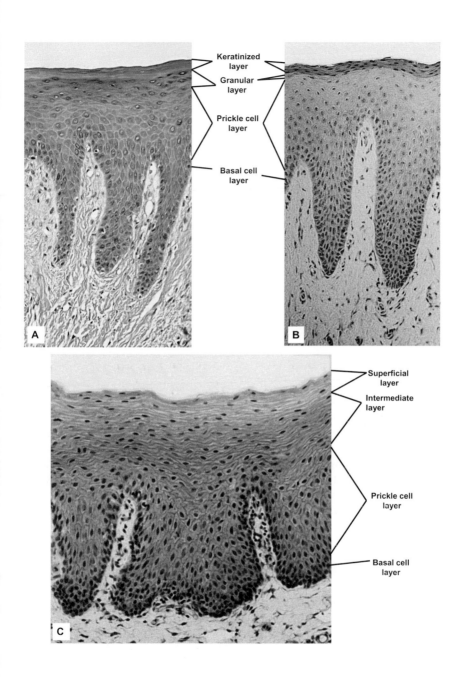

Keratinized
layer

Granular
layer

Prickle cell
layer

Basal cell
layer

Superficial
layer

Intermediate
layer

Prickle cell
layer

Basal cell
layer

A

B

C

The basal and prickle cell layers together constitute from half to two-thirds the thickness of the epithelium. The next layer consists of larger flattened cells containing small granules that stain intensely with hematoxylin. This layer is the *granular* layer, or *stratum granulosum*, and the granules are called *keratohyalin granules*. In some regions of the masticatory oral epithelium, such as the gingiva, these granules are difficult to discern under the light microscope. The surface layer is composed of very flat (squamous) cells, termed *squames*, that stain bright pink with eosin and do not contain any nuclei. This layer is the *keratinized layer* or *stratum corneum*. Other names sometimes used include *cornified layer* and *horny layer*. The pattern of differentiation of these cells is often termed *orthokeratinization*.

It is not unusual for masticatory mucosa (e.g., parts of the hard palate and much of the gingiva) to show a variation of keratinization known as *parakeratinization*. In parakeratinized epithelium (Fig. 3.1B), the surface layer stains for keratin, as described previously, but shrunken (or pyknotic) nuclei are retained in many or all of the squames. Keratohyalin granules may be present in the underlying granular layer, although usually fewer than in orthokeratinized areas, so that this layer is difficult to recognize in histological preparations. Parakeratinization is most commonly observed in the gingiva and is a normal event and does not imply disease; this is not true for epidermis, where parakeratinization may be associated with diseases such as psoriasis.

Another variant of keratinized or parakeratinized epithelium is sometimes seen when gingiva is prepared with stains such as Mallory's triple stain. The outermost squames of the keratinized (or parakeratinized) layer show a staining similar to that of deeper nucleated cells. Such an appearance is called *incomplete keratinization*, or incomplete parakeratinization, and it is suggested that the cells showing this pattern have become rehydrated by taking up fluid from the oral cavity. None of these variants of keratinization seems to have any pathologic significance in oral tissues.

### 3.1.2 Non-keratinization

The lining mucosa of the oral cavity, which is present on the lips, buccal mucosa, alveolar mucosa, soft palate, underside of the tongue, and floor of the mouth, has an epithelium that is usually non-keratinized (Fig. 3.1C). In many regions it is thicker than keratinized epithelium and shows a different ridge pattern at the connective tissue interface. Epithelium of the cheek, for example, may reach a thickness of more than 500 μm and has broader epithelial ridges than keratinized epithelium.

The basal and prickle cell layers of non-keratinized oral epithelium generally resemble those described for keratinized epithelium, although the cells of non-keratinized epithelium are slightly larger and the intercellular bridges or prickles are less conspicuous. For this reason, some people prefer to avoid the term *prickle cell layer* for non-keratinized epithelium. There are no sudden changes in the appearance of cells above the prickle cell layer in non-keratinized epithelium, and the outer half of the tissue is divided rather arbitrarily into two zones: intermediate *(stratum intermedium)* and superficial *(stratum superficiale)*. Schroeder (1981) refers to the latter layer as the *stratum distendum*, reflecting its mechanical flexibility. A granular layer is not present, and the cells of the superficial layer contain nuclei that are rarely shrunken or pyknotic. This layer does not stain intensely with eosin, as does the surface of keratinized or parakeratinized epithelium.

### 3.1.3 Variation of patterns of epithelial differentiation

Although the distribution of keratinized and non-keratinized epithelium in different anatomic locations is determined during embryologic development, there is often some variation of this basic pattern in adults. For example, the normally non-keratinized buccal mucosa develops a thin keratin layer, the *linea alba*, along the occlusal line as a result of mechanical irritation from chewing. The chemical irritation from the use of smokeless tobacco can also result in keratinization of non-keratinized buccal and labial mucosa ("tobacco keratosis"; Fig. 3.2A). Hyperkeratosis of non-keratinized oral epithelium may be physiologic, but it can also be associated with abnormal cellular changes that eventually lead to cancer of the squamous epithelium. Such hyperkeratotic lesions should be biopsied so that a diagnosis can be made. Similarly, the normal keratin layer of the palate may become greatly thickened in smokers, but such hyperkeratotic epithelium in other ways appears normal (Fig. 3.2B,C). In general, *hyperkeratosis* of oral epithelium that is normally keratinized represents a physiologic response of the epithelium to chronic physical irritation, similar to that occurring in callous formation on the palms and soles, or to chemical irritation, such as that from tobacco. The presence of inflammation in regions like the gingiva can reduce the degree of keratinization so that it appears parakeratinized or even non-keratinized. This change from one pattern of maturation to another, or the emphasis or depression of an existing trait, is usually reversible when the stimulus is removed.

## 3.2 EPITHELIAL PROLIFERATION AND TURNOVER

The oral epithelium, like other covering and lining epithelia, maintains its structural integrity by a process of continuous cell renewal in which cells produced by mitotic divisions in the deepest layers migrate to the surface to replace those that are shed (Nakamura et al., 2007). The cells of the epithelium can thus be considered to consist of two functional populations: a *progenitor population* (whose function is to divide and provide new cells) and a *maturing population* (whose cells are

**Figure 3.2**  Variations in keratinization. (A) Keratinization of non-keratinized buccal epithelium resulting from irritation by smokeless tobacco use. (B) Keratinization in normal palate. (C) Hyperkeratosis in hard palate as result of irritation by smoking.

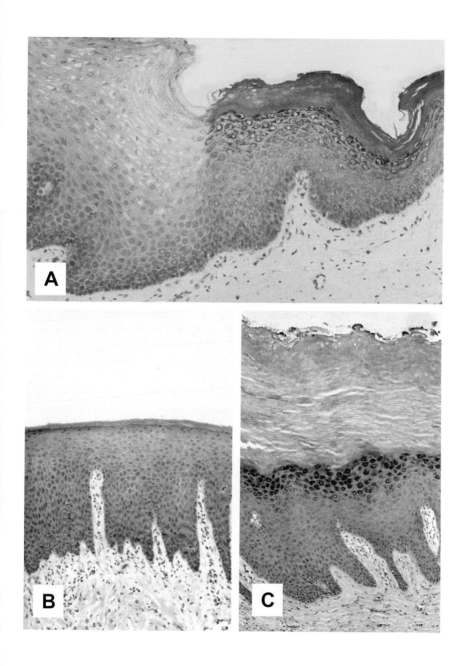

continually undergoing a process of differentiation or maturation to form a protective surface layer). These two important processes, proliferation and differentiation, are next considered in more detail.

The progenitor cells are situated in the basal layer in thin epithelia (e.g., the floor of the mouth) and in the lower two to three cell layers in thicker epithelia (cheeks and palate). Dividing cells tend to occur in clusters that are seen more frequently at the bottom of epithelial ridges than at the top. Studies on both the epidermis and the oral epithelium indicate that the progenitor compartment is not homogeneous but consists of two functionally distinct subpopulations of cells. A small population of progenitor cells cycles very slowly and is considered to represent stem cells, whose function is to produce basal cells and retain the proliferative potential of the tissue. The larger portion of the progenitor compartment is composed of amplifying cells, whose function is to increase the number of cells available for subsequent maturation.

Although they have no unique biochemical or ultrastructural features, oral keratinocyte progenitor stem cells have a number of identifying characteristics (Table 3.1). They are relatively small compared to other cells in these tissues and are $33.9 \pm 0.9\,\mu m$ in size (Izumi et al., 2007). Second, they express p75, a low-affinity neurotrophin receptor (Nakamura et al., 2007). p75 is a member of the Tumor Necrosis Factor family of receptors. It mediates cell survival, apoptosis, and intracellular signaling in neuronal tissues. p75 is expressed in the basal cell layer of the tips of the papillae and occasionally in the deep rete ridges of the buccal mucosa, whereas p75 is expressed in the basal cell layer of both the tips of the papillae and the deep rete ridges of the gingiva.

Progenitor stem cells have the capacity for long-term, error-free self-renewal with a high proliferative potential. In response to injury or when stimulated to proliferate, p75 expressing clones of progenitor stem cells divide into cells of different functions. One daughter resembles the original progenitor stem cell, and the other daughter forms a transient amplifying cell. New transient amplifying cells are

**Table 3.1**  Characteristics of oral keratinocyte progenitor stem cells.

| Characteristic | Reference |
| --- | --- |
| Found in well-protected, highly vascularized, and innervated areas | (Nakamura et al., 2007) |
| Small, 33.9 ± 0.9 μm in size | (Izumi et al., 2007; Nakamura et al., 2007) |
| Capacity for long-term, error-free self-renewal with a high proliferative potential | (Nakamura et al., 2007) |
| Higher *in vitro* proliferative capacity and clonal growth potential | (Nakamura et al., 2007) |
| High expression of p75, a low-affinity neurotrophin receptor | (Nakamura et al., 2007) |
| Low expression of Ki67, a marker for actively cycling cells indicating slow and infrequent cycling | (Nakamura et al., 2007) |
| Expression of integrin β1 | (Izumi et al., 2007; Nakamura et al., 2007) |
| Neurotrophin induces expression of keratin K13 but not K10 | (Nakamura et al., 2007) |
| Expression of peroxisome proliferator-activated receptor–gamma (PPAR-γ) | (Izumi et al., 2007) |

involved in the routine proliferative activities. Mature transient amplifying cells are capable of extensive expansion of the cell population. When finished, they undergo maturation or terminal differentiation. Because epithelial stem cells divide infrequently, they may be important in protecting the genetic information of the tissue, for DNA is most vulnerable to damage during mitosis.

Regardless of whether the cells are of the stem or amplifying type, cell division is a cyclic activity and is commonly divided into four distinct phases. The only phase that can be distinguished histologically is mitosis, which can be further subdivided into the recognizable stages of prophase, metaphase, anaphase, and telophase. After cell division, each daughter cell either recycles in the progenitor population or enters the maturing compartment.

**Table 3.2**  Epithelial turnover time in selected tissues.

| Tissue region | Median turnover time (days) |
|---|---|
| Small intestine | 4 |
| Buccal mucosa | 14 |
| Floor of mouth | 20 |
| Hard palate | 24 |
| Skin | 27 |

*Source:* Squier and Kremer (2001).

Epithelial cells in different tissues divide at greatly different rates. Apart from measuring the number of cells in division, it is also possible to estimate the time necessary to replace all the cells in the epithelium. This is known as *turnover time* of the epithelium and is derived from a knowledge of the time it takes for a cell to divide and pass through the entire epithelium.

Different techniques have led to a wide range of estimates of the rate of cell proliferation in the various epithelia; but, in general, epithelial turnover time is slower in the skin than in the oral mucosa which, in turn, is slower than the intestine (see Table 3.2). Regional differences in the patterns of epithelial maturation appear to be associated with the different turnover rates; for example, non-keratinized buccal epithelium turns over faster than keratinized palatal epithelium.

Cancer chemotherapeutic drugs act by blocking mitotic division of rapidly dividing cancer cells, as well as normal host cells. Normal host tissues that have a relatively short turnover time, such as blood cell precursors in bone marrow, intestinal epithelium, and oral epithelium, often are damaged by chemotherapeutic drugs. A significant number of patients taking chemotherapeutic drugs develop oral ulcers as a result of the breakdown of the overlying epithelium and thus experience pain and difficulty in eating, drinking, and maintaining oral hygiene.

Epithelial proliferation in oral mucosa, skin, and many other tissues is controlled by locally secreted peptide growth factors, or cytokines, including epidermal growth factor (EGF), keratinocyte growth factor (KGF), interleukin-1 (IL-1), and transforming growth factors (TGFs) α and β. These have antagonistic effects, so while EGF upregulates division, it is depressed by TGF-β. Cytokine activity is apparently modulated by families of proteins that mediate cell-to-cell (integrins) and cell-to-matrix adhesion (cadherins) in epithelia. Thus, integrins may interact with EGF receptors to amplify proliferation signals, whereas cadherins may reduce the cells' responsiveness to EGF (Müller et al., 2008).

Mitotic activity can also be affected by factors such as the time of the day, stress, and inflammation. For example, the presence of slight subepithelial inflammatory cell infiltration stimulates mitosis, whereas severe inflammation causes a marked reduction in proliferative activity. These effects probably represent the influence of different levels of proinflammatory cytokines and may be important when attempting to determine epithelial turnover in regions that are frequently inflamed, such as the dentogingival junction (see Chapter 6).

# 3.3 MOLECULAR AND CELLULAR ORGANIZATION OF ORAL EPITHELIUM

## 3.3.1 Molecular and cellular basis of differentiation

The genetic regulation of the transition from proliferation to differentiation is probably controlled by small non-coding RNAs (microRNAs; Yi et al., 2008) that promote exit from the cell cycle.

Epithelia differentiate according to their specific locations within the oral cavity and their related protective and immunologic functions (Gibbs and Ponec, 2000; Lindberg and Rheinwald, 1990). Cells of the basal layer are the least differentiated oral epithelial cells. They contain not only organelles commonly present in the cells of other tissues but also certain characteristic structures that identify them as epithelial cells and distinguish them from other cell types. These structures are the filamentous strands called *tonofilaments* and the intercellular bridges or desmosomes (Fig. 3.3B). Tonofilaments are fibrous proteins synthesized by the ribosomes and are seen as long filaments with a diameter of approximately 8 nm. They belong to a class of intracellular filaments called intermediate filaments and form an important structural component within the cell. Chemically, the filaments represent a class of intracellular proteins known as *cytokeratins*, which are characteristic constituents of epithelial tissues. When they become aggregated to form the bundles of filaments called *tonofibrils*, they can often be identified with the higher magnifications of the light microscope (Fig. 3.3A). One name often given to an epithelial cell because of its content of keratin filaments is *keratinocyte*. This serves to distinguish these epithelial cells from the non-keratinocytes that are described later.

There are a variety of markers that characterize keratinocytes, which are useful in delineating the mechanisms and extent of their differentiation (Table 3.3). Because of their ubiquity, keratins have become one of the more useful markers of epithelial differentiation.

The keratin family contains 20 different proteins that are useful as markers of differentiation (Lindberg and Rheinwald, 1990). Keratins are classified according to their mass, and the types of keratin present vary between different epithelia and even between the different cell layers of a single stratified epithelium. Those with the lowest molecular weight (40 kDa) are found in glandular and simple epithelia, those of intermediate molecular weight in stratified epithelia, and those with the highest molecular weight (67 kDa) in keratinized stratified epithelium. Keratin proteins K5, K6, K14, K16, and K17 are constitutively produced by cells of all stratified squamous epithelia in culture. K7, K8, K13, K18, and K19 production varies in cells from different regions of oral epithelium in culture. K1, K10, K13, and K19 production is useful as specific markers for assessing differentiation of epithelial cells. Keratins K1 and K10 are produced by suprabasal cells in keratinized oral epithelium, although occasionally they are present in the non-keratinized buccal epithelium;

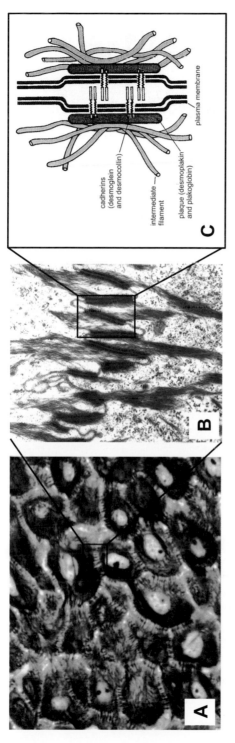

**Figure 3.3** Intercellular junctions. (A) Prickle cell layer in keratinized oral epithelium with intercellular bridges ("prickles") between adjacent cells. (B) Detail from A to show tonofibril attachment to desmosomes (box). (C) Diagram showing the detailed structure of a desmosome. ((B) from Squier and Finkelstein, 2003, Copyright Mosby; (C) modified from Dabelsteen, 1998. Reprinted with permission of SAGE Publications and Mosby.)

Within image C, labels read:
- cadherins (desmoglein and desmocollin)
- intermediate filament
- plaque (desmoplakin and plakoglobin)
- plasma membrane

**Table 3.3**  Markers of keratinocyte differentiation.

| Biochemical marker | Cell type | Reference |
|---|---|---|
| Profilaggrin, filaggrin | Keratinized epithelium | (Kautsky et al., 1995) |
| K1 | Keratinized epithelium | (Kautsky et al., 1995; Lindberg and Rheinwald, 1990) |
| K10 | Keratinized epithelium | (Gibbs and Ponec, 2000; Lindberg and Rheinwald, 1990) |
| K13 | Non-keratinized and keratinized epithelium | (Kautsky et al., 1995; Lindberg and Rheinwald, 1990) |
| K19 | Keratinized epithelium (basal cells) | (Kautsky et al., 1995; Lindberg and Rheinwald, 1990) |
| Involucrin | Non-keratinized and keratinized epithelium | (Gasparoni et al., 2004; Gibbs and Ponec, 2000; Lindberg and Rheinwald, 1990) |
| p75 | Oral keratinocyte progenitor stem cells | (Nakamura et al., 2007) |
| Ki67 | A marker for actively cycling cells | (Gibbs and Ponec, 2000; Nakamura et al., 2007) |
| Loricrin | A predominant protein of the cornified envelope in keratinocytes | (Gibbs and Ponec, 2000; Maestrini et al., 1996) |
| SPRR2 and SPRR3, small proline-rich proteins | Expression is strictly linked to keratinocyte terminal differentiation both *in vivo* and *in vitro* | (Gibbs and Ponec, 2000) (Lohman et al., 1997) |
| E-cadherin | Epithelial cells/ desmosomes | (Gasparoni et al., 2004) |
| Integrin β1 | Basal epithelial cells/ basal lamina | (Gasparoni et al., 2004; Izumi et al., 2007; Nakamura et al., 2007) |

this has been related to the ability of buccal mucosa to develop a keratinized surface as a result of mechanical or chemical irritation (Presland and Dale, 2000). K13 is produced by suprabasal cells in keratinized and non-keratinized oral epithelium, and K19, a 40 kDa protein, is produced by basal cells in non-keratinized oral epithelium and by junctional epithelium (see Chapter 6). K19 is also expressed by some human oral squamous cell carcinomas in culture.

Stratified epithelia possess a variety of cell surface carbohydrates that reveal differences during epithelial differentiation (Dabelsteen et al., 1991). Much of the research on both keratins and cell surface markers has focused on identifying changes indicative of aberrant maturation so as to provide early warning of disease processes such as cancer. It has also enabled distinction of the various types of epithelia making up the dentogingival junction (see Chapter 6).

An important property of any epithelium is its ability to function as a barrier, which depends to a great extent on the physical and chemical attachment between the epithelial cells. Cohesion between cells is provided by intercellular protein–carbohydrate complexes produced by the epithelial cells. In addition, there are modifications of the adjacent membranes of cells, the most common of which is the desmosome.

Desmosomes or *macula adherens* (Fig. 3.3B,C) are circular or oval areas of adjacent cell membranes, adhering by specialized intracellular thickenings known as *attachment plaques* and consisting of the proteins *desmoplakin* and *plakoglobin*. These link the intermediate filaments to the *cadherins*, a class of adhesive proteins that penetrate the membrane and enter the intercellular region of the desmosome. Apart from their role in providing mechanical adhesion between keratinocytes, desmosomes may also regulate signaling molecules concerned with epithelial proliferation and differentiation (Garrod and Chidgey, 2008). Adhesion between the epithelium and connective tissue is provided by *hemidesmosomes*, which are present on the basal membranes of cells of the basal layer (see Fig. 4.2). These also possess intracellular attachment plaques with tonofilaments inserted. Although the term hemidesmosome and its morphologic appearance suggest that this structure is half a desmosome, studies indicate that desmosomes and hemidesmosomes have different molecular constituents (compare Fig. 3.3B,C and Fig. 4.2).

The desmosomes, hemidesmosomes, and tonofilaments together represent a mechanical linkage that distributes and dissipates localized forces applied to the epithelial surface over a wide area. In some diseases, such as *pemphigus*, in which blistering of the epithelium occurs, there is a splitting of the epithelial layers to form bullous or vesicular lesions within the epithelium. This splitting is due to the breakdown of certain components of the desmosomal attachments, probably as a consequence of IgG auto-antibodies directed against the intercellular cadherin, *desmoglein* (Scully and Mignogna, 2008).

Two other types of connection are seen between cells of the oral epithelium: gap junctions and tight junctions. The gap junction, or *nexus*, is a region where membranes of adjacent cells run closely together, separated by only a small gap. There appear to be small interconnections between the membranes across these gaps. Such junctions may allow electrical or chemical communication between the cells and are sometimes called *communicating junctions*. They are seen only occasionally in oral epithelium. Even rarer in oral epithelium is the tight, or *occluding*, junction, where adjacent cell membranes are so tightly apposed that there is no intercellular space. In some epithelia these junctions may serve to seal off and compartmentalize the intercellular areas, but this is unlikely to occur in oral epithelium.

The major changes involved in cell differentiation in keratinized and non-keratinized oral epithelium are shown in the diagrams in Figure 3.4A,B. In both types of epithelia, the changes in cell size and shape are accompanied by a synthesis of more structural protein in the form of tonofilaments, the appearance of new organelles, and the production of additional intercellular material. There are, however, a number of changes that are not common to both epithelium and serve as distinguishing features. The cells of both epithelia increase in size as they migrate from the basal to the prickle cell layer, but this increase is greater in non-keratinized epithelium. There is also a corresponding syn-

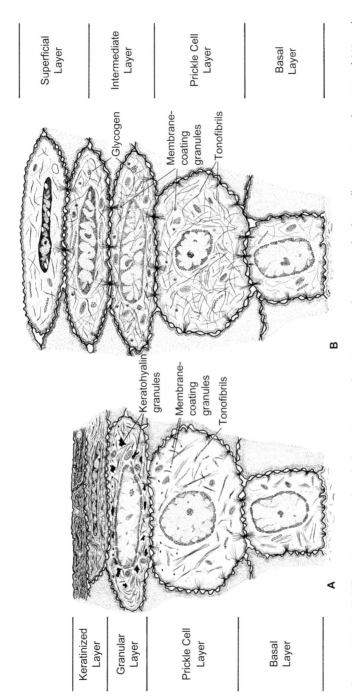

**Figure 3.4** Cell differentiation in oral epithelium. Diagram showing major changes involved in cell maturation in keratinized (A) and non-keratinized (B) oral epithelium.

thesis of tonofilaments in both epithelia, but whereas the tonofilaments in keratinized epithelium are aggregated into bundles to form tonofibrils (Fig. 3.5A), those in non-keratinized epithelium remain dispersed and so appear less conspicuous (Fig. 3.6A). We also know that the chemical structure of keratin filaments differs between layers so that various patterns of maturation can be identified by the keratins that are present.

In the upper part of the prickle cell layer there appears an organelle called the *membrane-coating* or *lamellate* granule. These granules are small, membrane-bound structures, about 250 nm in size, and contain glycolipid that probably originates from the Golgi system. In keratinized epithelium they are elongated and contain a series of parallel lamellae (Fig. 3.5A). In non-keratinized epithelium, by contrast, they appear to be circular with an amorphous core (Fig. 3.6A). As the cells move toward the surface, these granules become aligned close to the superficial cell membrane.

The next layer, called the *granular* layer in keratinized epithelium and the *intermediate* layer in non-keratinized epithelium, contains cells that have a greater volume but are more flattened than those of the prickle cell layer. In the upper part of this layer, in both keratinized and non-keratinized epithelia, the membrane-coating granules appear to fuse with the superficial cell membrane and to discharge their contents into the intercellular space. In keratinized oral epithelium and epidermis, the discharge of granule contents is associated with the formation of a lipid-rich permeability barrier that limits the movement of aqueous substances through the intercellular spaces of the keratinized layer. The granules seen in non-keratinized epithelium probably have a similar function, but the contents have a different lipid composition and do not form as effective a barrier as that in keratinized epithelia (see Chapter 8).

Cells in the superficial part of the granular layer develop a marked thickening on the inner (intracellular) aspect of cell membrane so as to form a cornified envelope that contributes to the considerable resistance of the keratinized layer to mechanical and chemical insult. One of the major constituents of this thickening is the protein *involucrin*, but *loricrin*

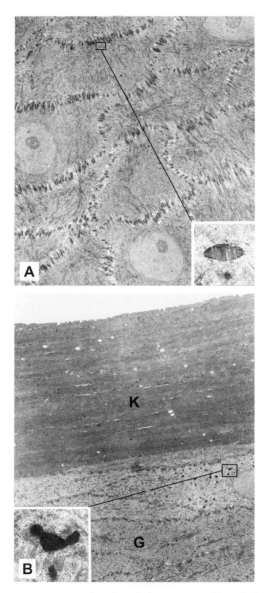

**Figure 3.5** Keratinized oral epithelium. (A) Prickle cells from keratinized gingival epithelium have elongated, lamellate membrane-coating granules (inset). (B) Irregularly shaped keratohyalin granules (inset) from the granular layer of gingival epithelium. ((A) (inset) and (B) from Squier and Finkelstein, 2003, Copyright Mosby.)

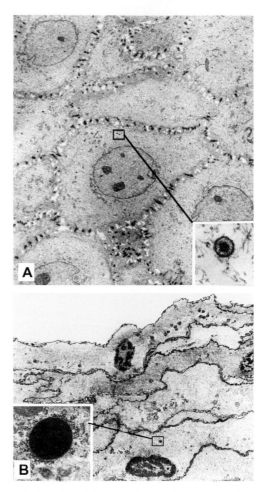

**Figure 3.6** Non-keratinized oral epithelium. (A) Prickle cells from non-keratinized buccal epithelium have circular membrane-coating granules with a dense core (inset). (B) Surface layer of non-keratinized oral epithelium that occasionally have keratohyalin granules (inset) that are regular in shape and surrounded by ribosomes. ((A) (inset) from Squier and Finkelstein, 2003, Copyright Mosby.)

and a number of *small proline-rich proteins (SPRs)* also contribute to the structure (Gibbs and Ponec, 2000; Presland and Dale, 2000). A similar, but less obvious, intracellular thickening consisting principally of involucrin is seen in the surface cells of non-keratinized epithelia. Despite their name, membrane-coating granules have nothing to do with this thickening. Involucrin is a useful marker in keratinized and non-keratinized epithelium (Table 3.3). The remaining events during epithelial differentiation are markedly different in keratinized and non-keratinized epithelia and so are described separately.

## Keratinization

The most characteristic feature of the granular layer of keratinized epithelium is the keratohyalin granules, which appear as basophilic granules under the light microscope and as electron-dense structures in the electron microscope (Fig. 3.5B). They are irregular in shape, usually between 0.5 and 1 nm in size, and are probably synthesized by the ribosomes that can be seen surrounding them. Keratohyalin granules are also intimately associated with tonofibrils, and they are thought to facilitate the aggregation and formation of cross-links between the cytokeratin filaments of the keratinized layer. For this reason, the protein making up the bulk of these granules has been named *filaggrin*, although the sulfur-rich protein, *loricrin*, is also present. Filaggrin is formed by phosphorylation of a precursor, profilaggrin; loricrin, profilaggrin, and filaggrin are all useful markers of epithelial differentiation (Table 3.3).

As the cells of the granular layer reach the junction with the keratinized layer, there is a sudden change in their appearance (Fig. 3.5B). All the organelles, including the nuclei and keratohyalin granules, disappear, and the cytokeratin filaments become associated with filaggrin, which is believed to facilitate their cross-linking by the formation of disulfide bonds. There is dehydration so that the cells of the keratinized layer are packed with filaments, are extremely flattened, and assume the form of hexagonal disks called *squames* (Fig. 3.7). Squames are lost (by the process of

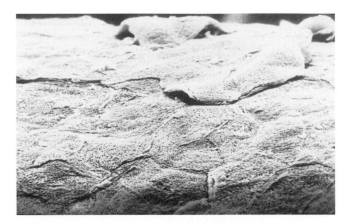

**Figure 3.7** Scanning electron micrograph of the flat, hexagonal-shaped surface cells (squames) of keratinized oral epithelium.

*desquamation*) and are replaced by cells from the underlying layers. This process may occur relatively rapidly so that an individual surface squame is shed in a matter of hours. The mechanism of desquamation is not well understood but probably represents a programmed process involving enzymatic degradation of desmosomal proteins and intercellular lipids by proteases and glycosidases (Milstone, 2004).

Rapid clearance of the surface layer is probably important in limiting the colonization and invasion of epithelial surfaces by pathogenic microorganisms, including the common oral fungus *Candida*.

The keratinized layer in the oral cavity may be composed of up to 20 layers of squames and is thicker than that in most regions of the skin except the soles and palms. The tightly packed cytokeratins within an insoluble and tough envelope make this layer resistant to mechanical and chemical damage.

## Non-keratinization

In non-keratinized oral epithelium, the events taking place in the upper cell layers are far less dramatic than those in keratinized epithelium (Fig. 3.6B). There is a slight increase in cell size in the intermediate cell layer as well as an accumulation of glycogen in cells of the surface layer. On rare occasions, keratohyalin granules can be seen at this level, but they differ from the granules in keratinized epithelium and appear as regular spherical structures surrounded by ribosomes but not associated with tonofilaments (Fig. 3.6B). Although they contain no filaggrin, loricrin is probably present and may contribute to the internal thickening of the cell membrane, already described. Keratohyalin granules sometimes remain in the surface cells where they may be evident in surface cytologic preparations.

In the superficial layer, there are few further changes. The cells appear slightly more flattened than in the preceding layers and contain dispersed tonofilaments and nuclei, the number of other cell organelles having diminished (Fig. 3.6B). The surface layer of non-keratinized epithelium thus consists of cells filled with loosely arranged filaments that are not dehydrated and represents a surface that is flexible and tolerant of both compression and distention.

# 3.4 NON-KERATINOCYTES IN THE ORAL EPITHELIUM

Sections of oral epithelium examined under the light microscope reveal the presence of a few cells that differ in appearance from other epithelial cells in having a clear halo around their nuclei (Fig. 3.8). Such cells have been termed *clear cells*, but it is obvious from ultrastructural and immunochemical studies that they represent a variety of cell types, including pigment-producing cells *(melanocytes)*, *Langerhans cells*, *Merkel cells*, and inflammatory cells (e.g., lymphocytes), which together make up as much as 10% of the cell population in the oral epithelium. All of these cells, except Merkel cells, lack desmosomal attachments to adjacent cells so that during histological processing the cytoplasm shrinks

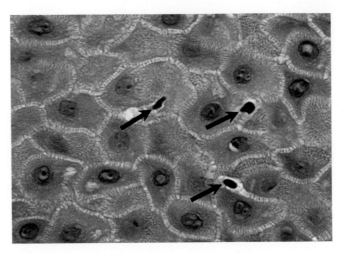

**Figure 3.8**   Clear cells (*arrows*) in prickle cell layer of oral epithelium are distinguished from adjacent keratinocytes by dark nuclei surrounded by a light halo.

around the nucleus to produce the clear halo. None of these cells contains the large numbers of tonofilaments and desmosomes seen in epithelial keratinocytes, and none participates in the process of maturation seen in oral epithelia; therefore, they are often collectively called *non-keratinocytes*.

## 3.4.1 Melanocytes and oral pigmentation

The color of the oral mucosa is the net result of a number of factors, including the vascularity of the underlying connective tissue, the presence and thickness of epithelial keratinization, and pigmentation. There are two types of pigmentation: endogenous, arising in specific cells as a result of normal physiologic processes, and exogenous, caused by foreign material introduced into the body either locally or systemically. The endogenous pigments most commonly contributing to the color of the oral mucosa are *melanin* and *hemoglobin* in red blood cells. Melanin is produced by specialized

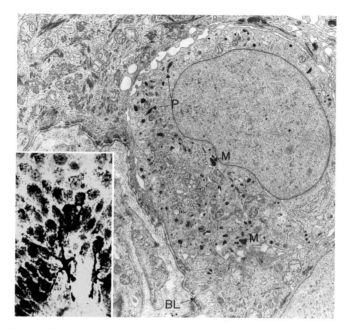

**Figure 3.9** Melanocyte in the basal layer of oral epithelium; electron micrograph of a cell situated adjacent to the basal lamina (BL) with premelanosomes (P) and melanosomes (M) present in the cytoplasm. Inset, melanocyte in oral epithelium stained by the Masson–Fontana silver method; the cell body is situated basally, although the dendritic processes extend well into the prickle cell layer.

pigment cells, called melanocytes, situated in the basal layer of the oral epithelium and the epidermis (Fig. 3.9 inset). Melanocytes arise embryologically from pluripotent cells of the neural crest ectoderm that can form melanoblasts. These cells proliferate and differentiate as they migrate from the neural crest to the basal layers of the epithelium, which they enter at about 11 weeks of gestation. There they continue to divide so as to maintain a self-reproducing population. They lack desmosomes and tonofilaments but possess long dendritic (branching) processes that extend between the keratinocytes, often passing through several layers of cells. Melanin is synthesized within the melanocytes as small structures called *melanosomes* (Fig. 3.9). These are formed initially from Golgi-derived vesicles or endosomes (premelanosomes) in which a series of protein filaments are formed. Melanins, which consist of copolymers of black and brown eumelanin or of red and yellow pheomelanin derived from tyrosine are laid down on the protein filaments. In albinism, melanosomes are formed, but there is a defect in the tyrosine pathway so pigment is not synthesized. Melanosomes are transported along microtubules within the melanocyte into the dendritic processes of the melanocytes from which they are injected or inoculated into the cytoplasm of adjacent keratinocytes. This probably involves specific receptors on the keratinocyte surface (Lin and Fisher, 2007).

Groups of melanosomes can often be identified under the light microscope in sections of heavily pigmented tissue stained with hematoxylin and eosin. These groups are referred to as melanin granules. In lightly pigmented tissues, the presence of melanin can only be demonstrated by specific histological and histochemical stains.

Both lightly and darkly pigmented individuals have the same number of melanocytes in any given region of skin or oral mucosa; color differences result from the relative activity of the melanocytes in producing melanin pigments and from the rate at which melanosomes are broken down within the keratinocytes. In persons with very heavy melanin pigmentation, cells containing melanin may be seen in the connective tissue. These cells are probably macrophages that have taken up melanosomes produced by melanocytes in the epithelium and are sometimes termed *melanophages*.

The regions of the oral mucosa where melanin pigmentation is most commonly seen clinically are the gingiva (Fig. 3.10), buccal mucosa, lips, hard palate, and tongue. Despite considerable individual variation, a direct relationship tends to be seen between the degrees of pigmentation in the skin and in the oral mucosa. Light-skinned persons rarely show any oral melanin pigmentation. In skin, melanocytes have an important role in protection against ionizing radiation, and melanin production is related to such exposure. This function is unlikely in oral mucosa, and their presence prob-

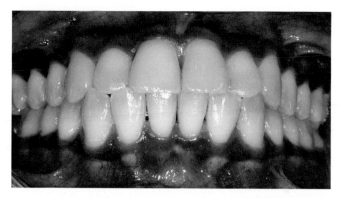

**Figure 3.10** Melanin pigmentation of the attached gingival in a dark-skinned individual. (Photograph courtesy of Dr. Georgia Johnson.)

ably reflects the programmed migration of melanocytes to ectodermal tissues. Mucosal irritation from smoking can result in increased melanin pigmentation (smoker's melanosis), which is seen in approximately 25% of smokers. Oral pigmentation may be increased as a result of systemic disease, the two most common being Addison's disease and Peutz–Jeghers' disease (Eisen, 2000).

Melanocytes are involved in the development of several pigmented lesions in the oral mucosa. *Oral melanotic macule* appears clinically similar to a freckle and microscopically shows increased production of melanin pigment without proliferation of melanocytes. It is harmless. A *nevus* (mole) is a benign proliferation of melanocytes and in the oral cavity that is not easy to distinguish clinically from melanoma. It should be completely removed. *Melanoma* is a malignant tumor of melanocytes. In the oral cavity, melanoma is rare, but prognosis is poor, with a 5-year survival rate of 10%–20%. Treatment is surgical removal.

One of the most common *exogenous* pigments is amalgam accidentally forced into the gingiva during placement of a restoration. This circumstance gives rise to patches of bluish gray discoloration known as amalgam tattoo. Certain metals (e.g., lead and bismuth) as well as carbon black, when present systemically, can give rise to pigmentation of the gingival margin (sometimes called *Burton's line*) and may be indicative of systemic poisoning.

## 3.4.2 Langerhans cells

The dendritic cell first described by Paul Langerhans in the epidermis in 1868 has only been well characterized in oral mucosa in the last 30 years. Functioning as a peripheral sentinel for the immune system, dendritic cells represent a group of antigen-presenting cells that include epidermal and oral epithelial Langerhans cells (Cutler and Jotwani, 2006). Langerhans cells are typically located in a suprabasal region in epidermis and oral epithelium, and because they lack desmosomal attachments to surrounding cells, appear as "clear cells" in histological sections. However, at the light microscope level, they can only be specifically identified with immunochemical markers to cell surface antigens, such as antibodies to human lymphocyte antigen DR (HLA-DR) and CD1a (Fig. 3.11 inset). Ultrastructurally, the Langerhans cell is characterized by the presence of a small rod- or flask-shaped granule, sometimes called the *Birbeck granule* (after the person who first described it under the electron microscope; Fig. 3.11).

It is believed that the highest numbers of Langerhans cells are found in non-keratinized mucosa of the soft palate, underside of tongue, lip, and vestibule, while lower numbers are found in the hard palate and gingiva. Such a distribution would accord with the higher permeability of non-keratinized tissue (see Chapter 8) and the proposed role of the Langerhans cell in antigen surveillance in the oral epithelium.

Langerhans cells first appear in the epithelium at the same time as, or just before, melanocytes, and they may be capable of limited division within the epithelium. Unlike melanocytes, they move in and out of the epithelium, and their source is likely to be the bone marrow. In the normal epithelium, Langerhans cells are associated with T-cell receptors on the keratinocyte surface and are oriented so that their dendrites extend toward the epithelial surface. This permits recognition and processing of antigenic material

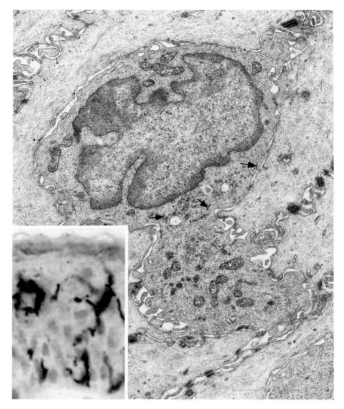

**Figure 3.11** Electron micrograph of a Langerhans cell in oral epithelium showing a convoluted nucleus lacking tonofilaments and desmosome attachments to adjacent cells but containing small rod- or flask-shaped granules (*arrows*). Inset, dendritic Langerhans cell in a suprabasal location stained for the cell surface antigen, CD1a.

that enters the epithelium from the external environment which is then presented to T lymphocytes. Langerhans cells migrate from epithelium into the lamina propria and to regional lymph nodes.

## 3.4.3 Merkel cells

The Merkel cell is situated in the basal layer of the oral epithelium and epidermis. Unlike the melanocyte and

Langerhans cell, it is not dendritic, although there may be surface protrusions or microvilli. Cytokeratin filaments are present in Merkel cells, and cytokeratin 20 has been claimed to represent a specific marker for Merkel cells in skin and oral mucosa. Occasional desmosomes link the Merkel cell to adjacent keratinocytes, and small hemidesmosomes are present at the basal lamina aspect. As a result, the cell does not shrink so as to appear as a "clear cell" in histological sections. The characteristic feature of Merkel cells is the presence of small membrane-bound vesicles in the cytoplasm, sometimes situated adjacent to a nerve fiber associated with the cell (Fig. 3.12). These granules may liberate a neuropeptide transmitter substance across the synapse-like junction between the Merkel cell and the nerve fiber and thus trigger an impulse. This arrangement is in accord with neurophysiologic evidence suggesting that Merkel cells are slowly

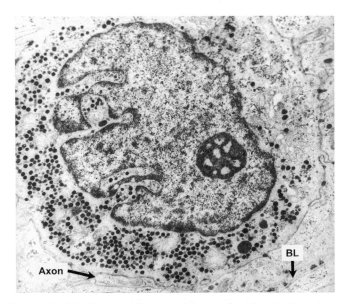

**Figure 3.12**  Merkel cell in basal layer of oral epithelium shows the cytoplasm filled with small, dense vesicles situated close to an adjacent unmyelinated nerve axon. Note location of basal lamina (BL). (Courtesy S.Y. Chen, reprinted from Squier and Finkelstein, 2003, Copyright Mosby.)

adapting mechanoreceptors and respond to touch. However, there have been reports of cells with characteristic granules that are positive for cytokeratin 20 and are located in the more superficial layers of palatal epithelium without an associated nerve fiber (Tachibana et al., 1998). Such cells may still have a sensory function, although an immunomodulating function has also been proposed for Merkel cells (Lucarz and Brand, 2007).

Although an origin of Merkel cells from neural crest ectoderm has been proposed, the presence of epithelial characteristics such as desmosomes and cytokeratin suggest that they may arise from division of keratinocytes (see Chapter 7, Section 7.1.).

### 3.4.4 Inflammatory cells and keratinocyte–non-keratinocyte interactions

When sections of epithelium taken from clinically normal areas of mucosa are examined microscopically, a number of inflammatory cells can often be seen in the nucleated cell layers. These cells are transient and do not reproduce themselves in the epithelium as the other non-keratinocytes do. The cell most frequently seen is the lymphocyte, although the presence of polymorphonuclear leukocytes and mast cells is not uncommon.

It is becoming evident that the association between non-keratinocytes and keratinocytes in skin and oral mucosa represents a subtle and finely balanced interrelationship in which keratinocytes are not bystanders. Keratinocytes have the capacity to secrete proinflammatory cytokines, including IL-1 and IL-8, that can lead to the recruitment of lymphocytes and polymorphonuclear leukocytes into the epithelium (Suchett-Kaye et al., 1998).

Lymphocytes are often associated with Langerhans cells, which are able to activate T lymphocytes. Thus, keratinocytes produce cytokines which modulate the function of Langerhans cells. In turn, the Langerhans cells produce cytokines such as IL-1, which can activate T lymphocytes so that they are capable of responding to antigenic challenge. IL-1 also increases the number of receptors to melanocyte-stimulating hormone in melanocytes and so can affect pigmentation. The influence of keratinocytes extends to the adjacent connective tissue, where cytokines produced in the epithelium can influence fibroblast growth and the formation of fibrils and matrix proteins.

# REFERENCES

Cutler, C.W., and Jotwani, R. (2006) Dendritic cells at the oral mucosal interface. J Dent Res 85:678–689.

Dabelsteen, E. (1998) Molecular biological aspects of acquired bullous diseases. Crit Rev Oral Biol Med 9(2):167–178.

Dabelsteen, E., Mandel, U., and Clausen, E. (1991) Cell surface carbohydrates are markers of differentiation in human oral epithelium. Crit Rev Oral Biol Med 2(4):493–507.

Eisen, D. (2000) Disorders of pigmentation in the oral cavity. Clin Dermatol 18:579–587.

Garrod, D., and Chidgey, M. (2008) Desmosome structure, composition and function. Biochim Biophys Acta 1778:572–587.

Gasparoni, A., Fonzi, L., Schneider, G.B., Wertz, P.W., Johnson, G.K., and Squier, C.A. (2004) Comparison of differentiation markers between normal and two squamous cell carcinoma cell lines in culture. Arch Oral Biol 49:653–664.

Gibbs, S., and Ponec, M. (2000) Intrinsic regulation of differentiation markers in human epidermis, hard palate and buccal mucosa. Arch Oral Biol 45:149–158.

Izumi, K., Tobita, T., and Feinberg, S.E. (2007) Isolation of human oral keratinocyte progenitor/stem cells. J Dent Res 86:341–346.

Kautsky, M.B., Fleckman, P., and Dale, B.A. (1995) Retinoic acid regulates oral epithelium differentiation by two mechanisms. J Invest Dermatol 104(4):546–553.

Lin, L., and Fisher, P.A. (2007) Melanocyte biology and skin pigmentation [Review]. Nature 445(7130):843–850.

Lindberg, K., and Rheinwald, J.G. (1990) Three distinct keratinocyte subtypes identified in human oral epithelium by their patterns of keratin expression in culture and in xenografts. Differentiation 45:230–241.

Lohman, F.P., Medema, J.K., Gibbs, S., Ponec, M., van de Putte, P., and Backendorf, C. (1997) Expression of the SPRR cornification genes is differentially affected by carcinogenic transformation. Exp Cell Res 231:141–148.

Lucarz, A., and Brand, G. (2007) Current considerations about Merkel cells. Eur J Cell Biol 86(5):243–251.

Maestrini, E., Monaco, A.P., McGrath, J.A., Ishida-Yamamoto, A., Camisa, C., Hovnanian, A., Weeks, D.E., Lathrop, M., Uitto, J., and Christiano, A.M. (1996) A molecular defect in loricrin, the major component of the cornified cell envelope, underlies Vohwinkel's syndrome. Nat Genet 13:70–77.

Milstone, L.M. (2004) Epidermal desquamation. J Dermatol Sci 36:131–140.

Müller, E.J., Williamson, L., Kolly, C., and Suter, M.M. (2008) Outside-in signaling through integrins and cadherins: a central mechanism to control epidermal growth and differentiation? J Invest Dermatol 128(3):501–516.

Nakamura, T., Endo, K., and Kinoshita, S. (2007) Identification of human oral keratinocyte stem/progenitor cells by neurotrophin receptor p75 and the role of neurotrophin/p75 signaling. Stem Cells 25:628–638.

Presland, R.B., and Dale, B.A. (2000) Epithelial structural proteins of the skin and oral cavity: function in health and disease. Crit Rev Oral Biol Med 11(4):383–408.

Schroeder, H.E. (1981) Differentiation of Human Oral Stratified Epithelia. S. Karger, Basel.

Scully, C., and Mignogna, M. (2008) Oral mucosal disease: pemphigus. Br J Oral Maxillofac Surg 46:272–277.

Squier, C.A., and Finkelstein, M.W. (2003) Oral mucosa. In: Ten Cate's Oral Histology, Development, Structure and Function (A. Nanci, ed.) pp. 329–375. Mosby, St. Louis, MO.

Squier, C.A., and Kremer, M.J. (2001) Biology of oral mucosa and esophagus. J Natl Cancer Inst Monogr 29:7–15.

Suchett-Kaye, G., Morrier, J.J., and Barsotti, O. (1998) Interactions between non-immune host cells and the immune system during periodontal disease: role of the gingival keratinocyte. Crit Rev Oral Biol Med 9:292–305.

Tachibana, T., Kamegai, T., Takahashi, N., and Nawa, T. (1998) Evidence for polymorphism of Merkel cells in the adult human oral mucosa. Arch Histol Cytol 61:115–124.

Yi, R., Poy, M.N., Stoffel, M., and Fuchs, E. (2008) A skin microRNA promotes differentiation by repressing "stemness." Nature 452:225–230.

# The interface between epithelium and connective tissue

The junction between the connective tissue and the overlying oral epithelium is seen in two-dimensional histological sections as an undulating interface at which papillae of the connective tissue interdigitate with the epithelial ridges (Fig. 4.1A). In three dimensions, the interface is seen to consist of connective tissue ridges, conical papillae, or both, projecting into the epithelium (Fig. 4.1B,C). The undulations increase the surface area of the interface and may provide better attachment and permit forces applied at the surface of the epithelium to be dispersed over a greater area of connective tissue. In this regard, it is notable that masticatory mucosa has the greatest number of papillae per unit area of mucosa; in lining mucosa, the papillae are fewer and shorter. The junction also represents an increased interface for metabolic exchange between the epithelium and the vasculature of the

*Human Oral Mucosa: Development, Structure, and Function.* Edited by
Christopher Squier and Kim A. Brogden.
© 2011 Christopher Squier and Kim A. Brogden. Published 2011 by
John Wiley & Sons, Inc.

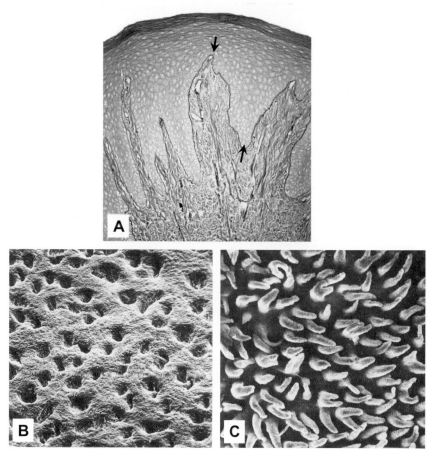

**Figure 4.1** (A) Gingival epithelium stained by the PAS method shows the basement membrane (*arrows*) and extensive interdigitation between epithelium and connective tissue. Scanning electron micrographs of gingival epithelium separated at this interface shows the circular orifices in the underside of the epithelium (B) into which fit the cone-shaped papillae of connective tissue (C). ((B) and (C) from Klein-Szanto and Schroeder, 1977, with permission from Wiley-Blackwell.)

connective tissue, for there are no blood vessels in the epithelium.

# 4.1 ORGANIZATION OF THE NORMAL INTERFACE

In routine hematoxylin and eosin stained histological sections of oral mucosa, the basement membrane between the epithelium and connective tissue appears as a structureless band, but it stains brightly with reagents such as periodic acid-Schiff (PAS) which detects glycogen, neutral mucosubstances, glycolipids, and phospholipids (Fig. 4.1A). Ultrastructurally, this region is described as the basal lamina or basal complex and is highly organized (Fig. 4.2). It consists of a layer of finely granular or filamentous material about 50 nm thick, the lamina densa, which runs parallel to the basal cell membranes of the epithelial cells but is separated from them by an apparently clear zone some 45 nm wide, the lamina lucida. Hemidesmosomes represent condensations of the proteins *bullous pemphigoid antigen* and *intermediate filament-associated protein* on the intracellular aspect of the basal cell plasma membrane (Dabelsteen, 1998). The cytokeratin (or intermediate) filaments loop into the *intermediate filament-associated protein*. Proteins belonging to the *integrin* family traverse the plasma membrane and enter the lamina lucida opposite hemidesmosomes, where they bind to laminin (Litjens et al., 2006). Hemidesmosomes occupy a greater proportion of the basal cell membrane in masticatory mucosa than in other regions, consistent with the concept of a stronger epithelial-connective tissue adhesion in this tissue (Grossman and Austin, 1983).

Inserted into the lamina densa are small loops of finely banded fibrils called *anchoring fibrils*. Collagen fibrils run through these loops and are thus interlocked with the lamina densa to form a flexible attachment. The lamina lucida contains glycoproteins, including the bullous pemphigoid antigen, which is a transmembrane component, probably associated with adhesion of the basal cell, and basement

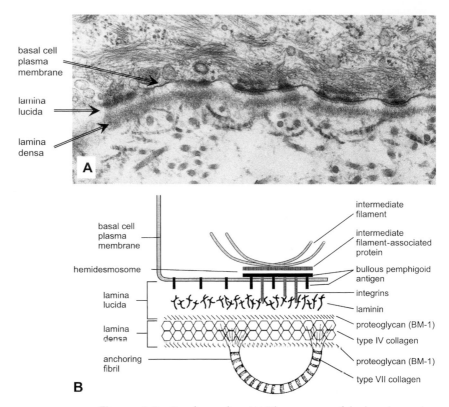

**Figure 4.2** Basal complex. (A) Ultrastructure of the basal complex in oral mucosa. (B) Diagram of the basal complex shows the fine structure of the junction between epithelium and connective tissue and identifies the location of principal molecular constituents of the junction. ((A) from Squier and Finkelstein, 2003, Copyright Mosby.)

membrane glycoprotein and laminin (Fig. 4.2B). The lamina densa contains type IV collagen arranged in a "chicken-wire" configuration. The proteoglycan heparan sulfate coats both surfaces of the lamina densa and may bind proteins, thus restricting their penetration. The anchoring fibrils consist of type VII collagen, and the collagens that run through the loops formed by the anchoring fibrils are type I and type III.

This complex arrangement of laminae and fibrils is clearly not a membrane in ultrastructural terms and is therefore more accurately called a basal complex or basal lamina. Seen under the light microscope with special stains, the basement membrane is a much thicker structure than the lamina lucida and lamina densa seen under the electron microscope. It probably includes some of the adjacent subepithelial collagen fibers (sometimes termed *reticulin* fibers), which also react with many of the histological basement membrane stains. It is now believed that all the basal lamina, except for its anchoring fibrils, is synthesized by the epithelium.

## 4.2 IMMUNE-MEDIATED SUBEPITHELIAL BLISTERING DISEASES (IMSEBDS)

The basal complex attaches the epithelium to connective tissue so that when the mucosa blisters, as in the lesions of pemphigoid, there is separation of the epithelium from connective tissue at the lamina lucida so as to create a subepithelial vesicle.

The basal lamina is the target of autoimmune disorders of oral mucous membranes (Scully and Lo Muzio, 2008). These disorders, called oral pemphigoid, consist of a family of chronic immune-mediated blistering diseases. These are "immune-mediated subepithclial blistering diseases" or IMSEBDs, and include bullous pemphigoid, pemphigoid (herpes) gestationis, cicatricial pemphigoid, dermatitis herpetiformis, and linear IgA disease. Lesions present as vesicles, bullae (blisters), or erosions on mucous membranes.

There are multiple target autoantigens involved in the pathogenesis of IMSEBDs (Scully and Lo Muzio, 2008). These include bullous pemphigoid antigen 2 (BPAg2 or BP180), bullous pemphigoid antigen 1 (BPAg1), laminin 5 (epiligrin), type VII collagen, the $\beta 4$ subunit of $\alpha 6\beta 4$ integrin, $\alpha 6$ integrin, and a 120-kDa protein found in gingiva. These autoantigens are in the epithelial basement membrane, in hemidesmosomes, or stratified squamous epithelium near the basal lamina.

The initiating factor in the pathogenesis of IMSEBDs is not known. Individuals with select genotypes and an association with HLA-DQB1*0301 or individuals exposed to select drugs like furosemide may be predisposed. Regardless, autoantibodies develop in the serum of patients with oral pemphigoid. These antibodies can be IgG with C3 or to a lesser degree IgA or IgM.

Lesions develop from an autoantibody-induced complement-mediated sequestration of polymorphonuclear leukocytes. These release cytokines and enzymes that detach the basal cells from the basement membrane zone. There may be some complement-mediated lysis of cells.

# REFERENCES

Dabelsteen, E. (1998) Molecular biological aspects of acquired bullous diseases. Crit Rev Oral Biol Med 9:162–178.

Grossman, E.S., and Austin, J.C. (1983) A quantitative electron microscope study of the desmosomes and hemidesmosomes in vervet monkey oral mucosa. J Periodontal Res 18:580–586.

Klein-Szanto, A.J.P., and Schroeder, H.E. (1977) Architecture and density of the connective tissue papillae of the human oral mucosa. J Anat 123:93–109.

Litjens, S.H., de Pereda, J.M., and Sonnenberg, A. (2006) Current insights into the formation and breakdown of hemidesmosomes. Trends Cell Biol 16:376–383.

Scully, C., and Lo Muzio, L. (2008) Oral mucosal diseases: mucous membrane pemphigoid. Br J Oral Maxillofac Surg 46:358–366.

Squier, C.A., and Finkelstein, M.W. (2003) Oral mucosa. In: Ten Cate's Oral Histology, Development, Structure and Function (A. Nanci, ed.) pp. 329–375. Mosby, St. Louis, MO.

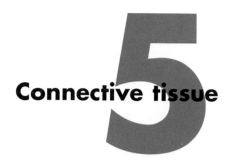

# Connective tissue

## 5.1 LAMINA PROPRIA

The connective tissue underlying the oral epithelium is called the lamina propria and can be divided into two layers: the superficial papillary layer (associated with the epithelial ridges or papillae) and the deeper reticular layer. The term *reticular* refers to the net-like arrangement of the collagen fibers; it has nothing to do with the so-called reticulin fibers, situated beneath the basal lamina.

The structural difference between these two layers is subtle and reflects the relative concentration and arrangement of the collagen fibers and of other components such as capillaries (Fig. 5.1A). In the papillary layer, collagen fibers are thin and loosely arranged, and many capillary loops are

*Human Oral Mucosa: Development, Structure, and Function.* Edited by Christopher Squier and Kim A. Brogden.
© 2011 Christopher Squier and Kim A. Brogden. Published 2011 by John Wiley & Sons, Inc.

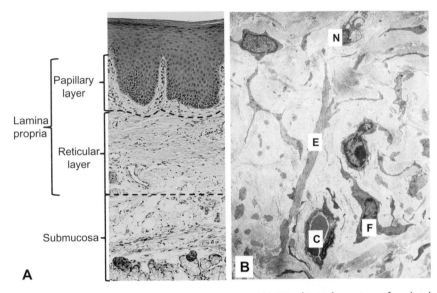

**Figure 5.1** Lamina propria. (A) Histological section of palatal mucosa showing approximate boundaries of the papillary and reticular layers in the lamina propria. (B) Electron micrograph of the lamina propria showing capillary (C), elastic fiber (E), nerve (N), and fibroblast (F) in the collagen. ((B) from Squier and Finkelstein, 2003, Copyright Mosby.)

present. By contrast, the reticular layer has collagen fibers arranged in thick bundles that tend to lie parallel to the surface plane.

The lamina propria consists of cells, blood vessels, neural elements, and fibers embedded in an amorphous ground substance (Fig. 5.1B). Like the overlying oral epithelium, it shows regional variation in the proportions of its constituent elements, particularly in the type, concentration, and organization of fibers.

### 5.1.1 Cells of the lamina propria

The lamina propria contains a variety of different cells: fibroblasts, macrophages, mast cells, and an array of inflammatory cells. A description of the major cells of the lamina propria can be found in Table 5.1.

**Table 5.1** Cell types in the lamina propria of oral mucosa.

| Cell type | Morphologic characteristics | Function | Location |
|---|---|---|---|
| Fibroblast | Stellate or elongated with abundant rough endoplasmic reticulum | Secretion of fibers and ground substance | Throughout lamina propria |
| Histiocyte | Spindle-shaped or stellate; often dark-staining nucleus; many lysosomal vesicles | Resident precursor of functional macrophage | Throughout lamina propria |
| Macrophage | Round with pale-staining nucleus; contains lysosomes and phagocytic vesicles | Mobile phagocytic cell; involved in antigen processing | Areas of chronic inflammation |
| Monocyte | Round with dark-staining kidney-shaped nucleus and moderate amount of cytoplasm | Phagocytic cell; blood-borne precursor of macrophage | Areas of inflammation |
| Mast cell | Round or oval basophilic granules staining metachromatically | Secretion of certain inflammatory mediators and vasoactive agents | Throughout lamina propria, often subepithelial |
| Polymorphonuclear leukocytes | Round with characteristic lobed nucleus; contains lysosomes and specific granules | Phagocytosis and cell killing | Areas of acute inflammation; may be present in epithelium |
| Lymphocyte | Round with dark-staining nucleus and scant cytoplasm with some mitochondria | Some lymphocytes participate in humoral or cell-mediated immune response | Areas of acute and chronic inflammation; may be present in epithelium |
| Plasma cell | Cartwheel nucleus; intensely pyroninophilic cytoplasm with abundant rough endoplasmic reticulum | Synthesis of immunoglobulins | Areas of chronic inflammation, often perivascularly |
| Endothelial cell | Normally associated with a basal lamina; contains numerous pinocytotic vesicles | Lining of blood and lymphatic channels | Throughout lamina propria |

## Fibroblasts

The principal cell in the lamina propria of oral mucosa is the fibroblast, which is responsible for the elaboration and turn-over of both fiber and ground substance. It thus plays a key role in maintaining tissue integrity.

Under the light microscope, fibroblasts are either cigar-shaped (fusiform) or star-shaped (stellate) with long processes that tend to lie parallel to bundles of collagen fibers and are not easily visible with the light microscope. Their nuclei contain one or more prominent nucleoli. Ultrastructurally, (Fig. 5.2A) fibroblasts have the characteristics of active synthetic cells, including numerous mitochondria, an extensive granular endoplasmic reticulum (which is often distended by its contents), a prominent Golgi complex, and numerous membrane-bound vesicles. Fibroblasts have a low rate of proliferation in adult oral mucosa except during wound healing, when their number increases as a result of fibroblast division in the adjacent uninjured tissues. It is now becoming apparent that they have varied roles depending on environmental demands. Fibroblasts can become "contractile" and participate in wound contraction, in which case they develop intracytoplasmic actin filaments. In certain disease states (e.g., the gingival overgrowth sometimes seen with phenytoin, calcium channel blockers such as nifedipine, and cyclosporine A, an immunosuppressant drug used in organ transplants), fibroblasts may secrete more ground substance than normal, and breakdown of type I collagen is reduced (Kataoka et al., 2005). Fibroblasts exhibit remarkable anatomic site specificity, evident in gene expression patterns, particularly among the HOX gene family (Rinn et al., 2008). Dependent on anatomic site, fibroblasts may have an important role in induction of overlying epithelia and development of fibrosis in wound healing as a result of interaction with other cells via cytokine growth factors, such as TGF-$\beta$ (Atamas, 2002).

## Macrophages

The fixed macrophage (*histiocyte*) is also a stellate or fusiform cell, and unless it is actively phagocytosing extracellular

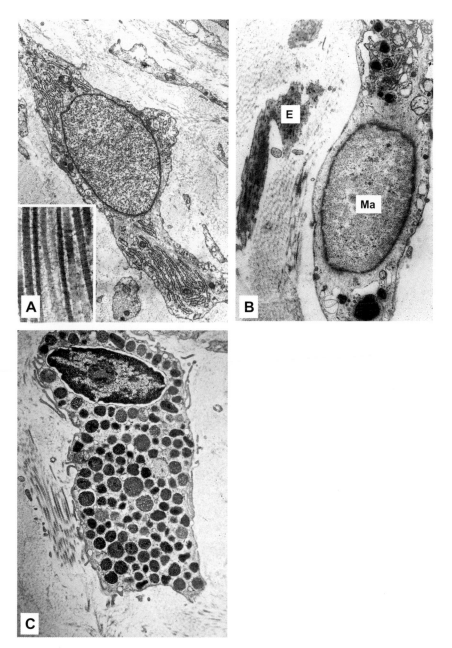

**Figure 5.2** Cells in lamina propria. (A) Fusiform-shaped fibroblast; the long processes tend to lie parallel to bundles of collagen fibers shown in the inset at high magnification. (B) Part of a macrophage (Ma) adjacent to elastic fibers (E). (C) Mast cell showing characteristic dense granules in cytoplasm. ((A) and (B) from Squier and Finkelstein, 2003, Copyright Mosby.)

debris, it may be difficult to distinguish from a fibroblast under the light microscope. Ultrastructurally, macrophages have smaller and denser nuclei and less granular endoplasmic reticulum than fibroblasts, and their cytoplasm contains membrane-bounded vesicles that can be identified as lysosomes (Fig. 5.2B).

The macrophage has a number of functions, the principal one being to ingest damaged tissue or foreign material in phagocytic vacuoles that fuse, intracytoplasmically, with lysosomes and initiate breakdown of these materials. The processing of ingested material by the macrophage may be important in increasing its antigenicity before it is presented to cells of the lymphoid series for subsequent immunologic response. Another important function is the production of cytokines and chemokines that stimulate fibroblast proliferation and collagen production necessary for repair (Atamas, 2002).

In the lamina propria of the oral mucosa, two special types of macrophages can be specifically identified: the *melanophage* and the *siderophage*. The melanophage, which is common in pigmented oral mucosa, is a cell that has ingested melanin granules extruded from melanocytes within the epithelium. The siderophage is a cell that contains hemosiderin derived from red blood cells that have been extravasated into the tissues as a result of mechanical injury. This material can persist within the siderophage for some time, and the resultant brownish color appears clinically as a bruise.

## Mast cells

The mast cell is a large spherical or elliptical mononuclear cell (Fig. 5.2C). Its nucleus is small relative to the size of the cell and in histologic preparations is frequently obscured by the large number of intensely staining granules that occupy its cytoplasm. These granules stain with certain basic dyes such as methylene blue because of the presence of heparin within the granules. In humans, the principal contents of the granules are histamine and heparin and cytokines such as tumor necrosis factor alpha (TNF-α) and interleukins.

Mast cells are primarily located adjacent to the basement membrane of endothelial cells and nerves in the connective tissue of oral mucosa. Their migration is influenced by synthesis of mast cell growth factor (MGF) by enodothelial cells and keratinocytes (Walsh, 2003). Because these cells are frequently found in association with small blood vessels, it has been suggested that they play a role in the development of inflammation and in the shift from acute to chronic inflammation.

*Inflammatory cells*

Histologically, the lymphocyte and plasma cell may be observed in small numbers scattered throughout the lamina propria, but apart from such specialized regions as the lingual tonsil, other inflammatory cells are found in significant numbers only in connective tissue, either following an injury (e.g., a surgical incision) or as part of a disease process. When inflammatory cells are present in significant numbers, they influence the behavior of the overlying epithelium by releasing cytokines.

As in other parts of the body, the type of inflammatory cell is dependent on the nature and duration of the injury. In acute conditions, polymorphonuclear leukocytes are the dominant cell type, whereas in more chronic conditions (e.g., periodontal disease), the majority of these cells are T lymphocytes with lesser amounts of macrophages, monocytes, B lymphocytes, plasma cells, and dendritic Langerhans cells. The recruitment of polymorphonuclear leukocytes and macrophages represents an important component of the innate immune response to infection in the mucosa (Dongari-Bagtzoglou and Fidel, 2005).

## 5.1.2 Fibers and ground substance of lamina propria

The lamina propria contains a three-dimensional network of fibers arranged in groups and ground substance composed of water, glycoproteins, and proteoglycans and serum-derived proteins. There are two major types of fibers, collagen and elastin, together with fibronectin.

## Collagen

Currently, 28 different types of collagen composed of at least 46 distinct polypeptide chains have been identified (Shoulders and Raines, 2009). Collagen is typically organized as three parallel alpha polypeptide strands coiled in a helical conformation around each other. The individual collagen triple helices assemble in a complex, hierarchical manner that ultimately leads to the macroscopic fibers and networks observed in tissue, bone, and basement membranes. Variations in the assembly of these helices and the proportion of non-helical sequences gives rise to the different types of collagen which have different structure and function. The alignment of helices in collagens I, II, III, and V gives rise to fibrils that have a characteristic 64 nm banding pattern in electron microscope preparations (Fig. 5.2A). The location and function of the types of collagen that are present in oral mucosa are summarized in Table 5.2.

## Elastic fibers

The main components of elastic fibers are elastin and microfibrils. Elastin makes up the bulk of the mature fiber and is responsible for the elastic properties of the fiber. Microfibrils consist mainly of fibrillin, a glycoprotein, but also contain or are associated with proteins such as microfibril associated glycoproteins (MAGPs), fibulins, and the Elastin Microfibril Interface Located Protein (EMILIN) (Wagenseil and Mecham, 2007).

Microfibrils were thought to facilitate alignment of elastin monomers prior to cross-linking by lysyl oxidase, but other proteins and fibroblasts are involved (Wagenseil and Mecham, 2007). Initially, elastic fibers consist entirely of aggregates of microfibrils, each 10–20 nm in diameter. As they mature, however, elastin is laid down within the microfibril matrix as a granular material until it becomes the pre-

**Table 5.2**  Structure, distribution, and function of collagens in oral mucosa.

| Structure | Collagen type | Distribution and function |
|---|---|---|
| Fibrillar | I | Abundant in lamina propria of oral mucosa |
| | III | Present around blood vessels. Forms reticular fibers |
| | VII | Form anchoring fibrils at basal lamina |
| Microfibrillar | V | Present in basal laminae |
| Fibril-associated collagen with interrupted triple helices (FACIT) | XII, XIV, XIX, XX | Facilitates fiber interactions in connective tissue, including basal laminae and matrix attachment |
| Network or mesh | IV, VI | Structural component of basal laminae; facilitates attachment of cells to matrix |
| Membrane-associated collagen with interrupted triple helices (MACIT) | XIII, XVII | Facilitates cell-to-cell and cell-to-matrix attachment; found in hemidesmosomes |
| Multiple interrupted triple helix domains (MULTIPLEXIN) | XV, XVIII | Endothelial cell basal lamina; proteolysis releases endostatins which are potent anti-angiogenic factors |

*Source:* Shoulders and Raines (2009).

dominant component, accounting for more than 90% of the fiber (Fig. 5.2B).

When stained with aldehyde fuchsin, orcein, or Weigert's elastic stain, elastic fibers can be seen in most regions of the oral mucosa, but they are more abundant in the flexible lining mucosa, where they function to restore tissue form after stretching. Unlike collagen fibers, elastic fibers branch and anastomose and run singly rather than in bundles.

### 5.1.3 Ground substance

Although the ground substance of the lamina propria appears by both light and electron microscopy to be amorphous; at the molecular level it consists of heterogeneous protein–carbohydrate complexes permeated by tissue fluid. Chemically, these complexes can be subdivided into two distinct groups: proteoglycans and glycoproteins.

The proteoglycans consist of a polypeptide core to which glycosaminoglycans chains (GAGs; consisting of hexose and hexuronic acid residues) are attached. In the oral mucosa, the proteoglycans are represented by hyaluronan (which can aggregate with the proteoglycan monomers, aggrecan and versican to form hydrated gels), heparan sulfate (including agrin and perlecan that are present in basal laminae), biglycan and decorin (small proteoglycans involved in regulation of collagen fibril and matrix assembly), decorin and fibromodulin that bind to collagen, glypican, a membrane-bound proteoglcyan, and syndecan and CD44, which are transmembrane proteoglycans. Proteoglycans in the matrix are different from those associated with the cell surface, and interaction between them and with cell surface molecules (e.g., integrins) are probably important in modulating the behavior and function of cells; thus membrane -bound and transmembrane proteoglycans can bind growth factors. Glycoproteins consist of branched polypeptide chains to which only a few simple hexoses are attached. Several of these molecules, such as fibronectin and tenascin, play a role in binding cells to matrix proteoglycans and collagen.

## 5.2 BLOOD SUPPLY

The blood supply of the oral mucosa is extremely rich and is derived from arteries that run parallel to the surface in the submucosa or, when the mucosa is tightly bound to underlying periosteum and a submucosa is absent, in the deep part of the reticular layer. These vessels give off progressively smaller branches that anastomose with adjacent vessels in the reticular layer before forming an extensive

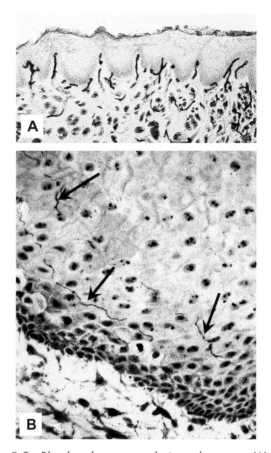

**Figure 5.3** Blood and nerve supply in oral mucosa. (A) Buccal mucosa stained to show the relationship of capillaries in the lamina propria and overlying epithelium. (B) Intraepithelial nerves (*arrows*) running between the cells of buccal epithelium. ((A) (Courtesy of G. Zoot) and (B) (courtesy of J. Linder) from Squier and Finkelstein, 2003, Copyright Mosby.)

capillary network in the papillary layer. From this network, capillary loops pass into the connective tissue papillae and come to lie close to, but never enter, the basal layer of the epithelium (Fig. 5.3A). The concentration of capillaries in oral mucosa is much greater than in skin, where capillary loops are found only in association with hair follicles, and this may explain the deeper color of oral mucosa.

Regional modifications occur in this basic pattern. For example, in the cheek, a single capillary loop passes into each papilla, but in the tongue, each filiform papilla receives a variable number of capillaries; in the larger fungiform and circumvallate papillae, arterioles reach into them before giving off capillary loops. In tissues such as the cheek, where the connective tissues may undergo extensive deformation, the arterioles follow a tortuous path and show more extensive branching.

Blood from the capillary beds is collected by a series of venules in the reticular layer, which connect with veins beneath the mucosa. Almost all the venous return is eventually carried by the internal jugular vein. Lymphatic capillaries are present in the lamina propria and arise as blind vessels in the papillae that drain into larger vessels in the submucosa. All the lymphatic vessels ultimately drain into the deep cervical lymph nodes.

Blood flow through the oral mucosa is greatest in the gingiva, but in all regions of the oral mucosa, it is greater than in the skin at normal temperatures. The extent to which inflammation in the gingiva, which is almost inevitably present, may be responsible for this greater flow is uncertain. Microorganisms and microbial by-products pass through the highly permeable junctional epithelium and enter the lamina propria. These microbial antigens stimulate local venules to express ELAM-1, ICAM-1, LFA-3, and VCAM-1 that attracts T cells via by their selectin and integrin surface receptors. This facilitates leukocyte trafficking, even in health.

Unlike the skin, which plays a role in temperature regulation, human oral mucosa lacks arteriovenous shunts, but it does have rich anastomoses of arterioles and capillaries, which undoubtedly contribute to its ability to heal more rapidly than skin after injury.

## 5.3 NERVE SUPPLY

The oral mucous membrane is densely innervated so that it can monitor all substances entering the oropharynx. A rich innervation also serves to initiate and maintain a wide variety of voluntary and reflexive activities involved in mastication, salivation, swallowing, gagging, and speaking. The nerve supply to the oral mucous membrane is therefore predominantly sensory.

The efferent supply is autonomic, supplies the blood vessels and minor salivary glands, and may also modulate the activity of some sensory receptors. The nerves arise mainly from the second and third divisions of the trigeminal nerve; but afferent fibers of the facial (VII), glossopharyngeal (IX), and vagus (X) nerves are also involved. The sensory nerves lose their myelin sheaths and form a network in the reticular layer of the lamina propria that terminates in a subepithelial plexus.

The sensory nerves terminate in both free and organized nerve endings. Free nerve endings are found in the lamina propria and within the epithelium, where they are frequently associated with Merkel cells (see Fig. 3.12). Apart from the nerves associated with Merkel cells, there are intraepithelial nerve endings that have a sensory function. Such nerves are not surrounded by Schwann cells as in connective tissue but run between the keratinocytes (which may ensheath the nerves and so form a mesaxon). These nerves terminate as simple endings in the middle, or upper, layers of the epithelium (Fig. 5.3B).

Within the lamina propria, organized nerve endings are usually found in the papillary region. They consist of groups of coiled fibers surrounded by a connective tissue capsule. These specialized endings have been grouped according to their morphology as *Meissner's* or *Ruffini's corpuscles, Krause's bulbs*, and the mucocutaneous end organs. The density of sensory receptors is greater in the anterior part of the mouth than in the posterior region, with the greatest density where the connective tissue papillae are most prominent.

The primary sensations perceived in the oral cavity are temperature, touch, pain, and taste. Although specialized nerve endings are differentially sensitive to particular modalities (e.g., Krause's bulbs appear to be most sensitive to cold stimuli and Meissner's corpuscles to touch), there is no evidence that a specific morphological form of receptor is responsible for detecting only one type of stimulus. It is likely, however, that each modality is served by specific fibers associated with each termination (see below).

Sensory nerve networks are more developed in the oral mucosa lining the anterior than the posterior regions of the mouth, and this pattern is paralleled by the greater sensitivity of this region to a number of modalities. For example, touch sensation is most acute in the anterior part of the tongue and hard palate. By comparison, the sensitivity of the fingertips falls between those of the tongue and the palate. Touch receptors in the soft palate and oropharynx are important in the initiation of swallowing, gagging, and retching. Similarly, temperature reception is more acute in the vermilion border of the lip, at the tip of the tongue, and on the anterior hard palate than in more posterior regions of the oral cavity. The detection of pain is complex but is becoming better understood. It appears to be initiated by stimuli which act on free nerve endings of two classes of nociceptors — medium-sized myelinated nerves that transmit acute or "fast" pain and small-diameter unmyelinated fibers that respond to poorly localized or "slow" pain (Basbaum et al., 2009). The acute nociceptors respond to heat above 43°C and below 10–12°C as pain and to chemical agents such as capsaicin, which are interpreted as "hot." These nociceptors also respond to an array of endogenous factors produced by tissue damage and inflammation, such as serotonin, histamine, glutamate, bradykinin, and various cytokines and chemokines.

## 5.3.1 Taste and taste buds

Taste bud cells, together with Merkel cells, are the only truly specialized sensory cells in the oral mucosa. Although some taste buds lie within the epithelium of the soft palate and pharynx, most are found in the fungiform, foliate, and circumvallate papillae of the tongue (see Figs. 5.4 and 6.2, 6.3, 6.4).

Histologically, the taste bud is a barrel-shaped structure composed of 30–80 spindle-shaped cells (see Fig. 5.4B,C). The apical ends of these cells are tightly joined together by

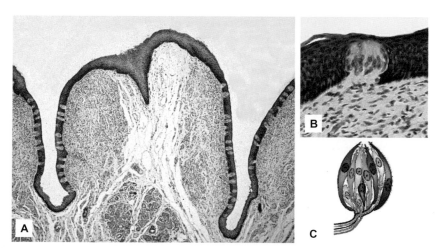

**Figure 5.4** Taste buds. (A) The non-keratinized epithelium of foliate papilla contain numerous taste buds situated laterally. (B) Histological section showing the barrel shaped structure of a taste bud. (C) Diagram to illustrate the concept that different receptor cells within a taste bud respond to different modalities conveyed by a nerve associated with the cell. ((C) Reprinted with permission from Macmillan Publisher's Ltd; Chandrashekar et al., 2006.)

junctional complexes, somewhat like those in intestinal mucosa. The initial events stimulating sensation of taste appear to involve the amorphous material within the taste pits and the microvilli of constituent cells that project into those pits. At their bases, the cells are separated from underlying connective tissue by the basement membrane, whereas their apical ends terminate just below the epithelial surface in a taste pit that communicates with the surface through a small opening, the taste pore. Taste bud cells are continually being replaced, and their maintenance depends on a functional gustatory nerve.

It is now established that the five taste modalities, sweet, salty, sour, bitter, and umami (or savory) are detected by different receptor cells within a taste bud (Fig. 5.4C), and the appropriate information is conveyed by a nerve associated with the cell (Chandrashekar et al., 2006). The same range of modalities are detected in taste buds wherever they occur in the oral cavity so that there is no regional specificity of taste. Taste stimuli are probably generated by the binding of molecules onto specific G-protein-coupled receptors on the surface of the taste bud cells which activates intracellular messengers. The change in membrane polarization that follows stimulates release of transmitter substances which, in turn, stimulate unmyelinated afferent fibers of the glossopharyngeal nerve (IX), which surround the lower half of the taste cells.

It has been suggested recently that there is a "fat" taste in addition to the modalities for sweet, salty, bitter, sour, and unami. In rodents, lipases secreted by the lingual papillae will liberate free fatty acids from long chain fatty acids that then bind to specific receptors on taste bud cells Gaillard et al. (2008), but it is uncertain whether such a mechanism is operative in humans.

The finding that the same region of the brain is activated by water as by salt and sweet (de Araujo et al., 2003) suggest that there may be receptors in the oral mucosa that respond to the "taste" of water and signal the satisfaction of thirst. This sensation may involve the standard taste receptors, and in particular the salty receptor, which may represent water by decreased firing when water is placed on the tongue.

## REFERENCES

de Araujo, I.E., Kringelbach, M.L., Rolls, E.T., and McGlone, F.J. (2003) Human cortical responses to water in the mouth, and the effects of thirst. Neurophysiology 90:1865–1876.

Atamas, S.P. (2002) Complex cytokine regulation of tissue fibrosis. Life Sci 27:631–643.

Basbaum, A.I., Bautista, D.M., Scherrer, G., and Julius, D. (2009) Cellular and molecular mechanisms of pain. Cell 139:267–284.

Chandrashekar, J., Hoon, M.A., Ryba, N.J.P., and Zuker, C.S. (2006) The receptors and cells for mammalian taste. Nature 444:288–294.

Dongari-Bagtzoglou, A., and Fidel, P.L. Jr. (2005) The host cytokine responses and protective immunity in oropharyngeal candidiasis. J Dent Res 84:966–977.

Gaillard, D., Passilly-Degrace, P., and Besnard, P. (2008) Molecular mechanisms of fat preference and overeating. Ann N Y Acad Sci 1141:163–175.

Kataoka, M., Kido, J., Shinohara, Y., and Nagata, T. (2005) Drug-induced gingival overgrowth — a review. Biol Pharm Bull 28:1817–1821.

Rinn, J.L., Wang, J.K., Liu, H., Montgomery, K., van de Rijn, M., and Chang, H.Y. (2008) A systems biology approach to anatomic diversity of skin. J Invest Dermatol 128:776–782.

Shoulders, M.D., and Raines, R.D. (2009) Collagen structure and stability. Annu Rev Biochem 78:929–958.

Squier, C.A., and Finkelstein, M.W. (2003) Oral mucosa. In: Ten Cate's Oral Histology, Development, Structure and Function (A. Nanci, ed.) pp. 329–375. Mosby, St. Louis, MO.

Wagenseil, J.E., and Mecham, R.P. (2007) New insights into elastic fiber assembly. Birth Defects Res C Embryo Today 81:229–240.

Walsh, L.J. (2003) Mast cells and oral inflammation. Crit Rev Oral Biol Med 14:188–198.

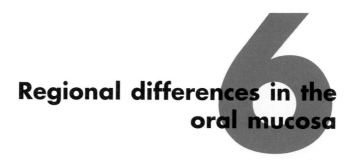

# Regional differences in the oral mucosa

## 6.1 STRUCTURAL VARIATIONS IN DIFFERENT REGIONS

The range of regional variation seen in oral mucosa is, if we exclude appendages such as nails and hair, even greater than that seen in skin. This range includes differences not only in the composition of the lamina propria, form of the interface between epithelium and connective tissue, and type of surface epithelium, but also in the nature of the submucosa and how the mucosa is attached to underlying structures. These regional differences are considered to represent functional adaptations, and the mucosa is consequently divided into three main types: masticatory, lining, and specialized. The regions occupied by each type have been illustrated in Figure 2.1. A summary of the mucosal organization within the various anatomic regions is given in Table 6.1, and a

*Human Oral Mucosa: Development, Structure, and Function.* Edited by Christopher Squier and Kim A. Brogden.
© 2011 Christopher Squier and Kim A. Brogden. Published 2011 by John Wiley & Sons, Inc.

**Table 6.1** Structure of the mucosa in different regions of the oral cavity.

| Region | Mucosa | | Submucosa |
|---|---|---|---|
| | **Covering epithelium** | **Lamina propria** | |
| Lining mucosa | | | |
| Soft palate | Thin (150 μm), non-keratinized stratified squamous epithelium; some taste buds present | Thick with numerous short papillae; elastic fibers forming an elastic lamina; highly vascular with well-developed capillary network | Diffuse tissue containing numerous minor salivary glands |
| Ventral surface of tongue | Thin, non-keratinized, stratified squamous epithelium | Thin with numerous short papillae and some elastic fibers; a few minor salivary glands, capillary network in subpapillary layer | Thin and irregular, where absent, mucosa is bound to connective tissue surrounding tongue musculature |
| Floor of mouth | Very thin (100 μm), non-keratinized stratified squamous epithelium | Short papillae; some elastic fibers; extensive vascular supply with short anastomosing capillary loops | Loose fibrous connective tissue containing fat and minor salivary glands |
| Alveolar mucosa | Thin, non-keratinized stratified squamous epithelium | Short papillae, connective tissue containing many elastic fibers; capillary loops close to the surface | Loose connective tissue, containing thick elastic fibers attaching it to periosteum of alveolar process; minor salivary glands |
| Labial and buccal mucosa | Very thick (500 μm), non-keratinized stratified squamous epithelium | Long, slender papillae; dense fibrous connective tissue containing collagen and some elastic fibers; rich vascular supply giving off anastomosing capillary loops into papillae | Mucosa firmly attached to underlying muscle by collagen and elastin; dense collagenous connective tissue with fat, minor salivary glands, some sebaceous glands |

| | Epithelium | Lamina propria | Submucosa/attachment |
|---|---|---|---|
| Lips: vermilion zone | Thin, orthokeratinized, stratified squamous epithelium | Numerous narrow papillae; capillary loops close to surface in papillary layer | Mucosa firmly attached to underlying muscle; some sebaceous glands in vermilion border, minor salivary glands and fat in intermediate zone |
| Lips: intermediate zone | Thin, parakeratinized, stratified squamous epithelium | Long irregular papillae; elastic and collagen fibers in connective tissue | |
| Masticatory mucosa | | | |
| Gingiva | Thick (250 μm), orthokeratinized or parakeratinized, stratified squamous epithelium often showing stippled surface | Long, narrow papillae, dense collagenous connective tissue; long capillary loops with numerous anastomoses | No distinct layer, mucosa firmly attached by collagen fibers to cementum and periosteum of alveolar process ("mucoperiosteum") |
| Hard palate | Thick, orthokeratinized (parakeratinized, in parts), stratified squamous epithelium thrown into transverse palatine ridges (rugae) | Long papillae; thick, dense collagenous tissue, especially under rugae; moderate vascular supply with short capillary loops | Dense collagenous connective tissue attaching mucosa to periosteum ("mucoperiosteum"), fat, and minor salivary glands are packed into connective tissue in regions where mucosa overlies lateral palatine neurovascular bundles |
| Specialized mucosa | | | |
| Dorsal surface of tongue | Thick, keratinized, and non-keratinized, stratified squamous epithelium forming three types of papillae, some bearing taste buds | Long papillae; minor salivary glands in posterior portion; rich innervations, particularly near taste buds; capillary plexus in papillary layer, large vessels lying deeper | No distinct layer; mucosa is bound to connective tissue surrounding musculature of tongue |

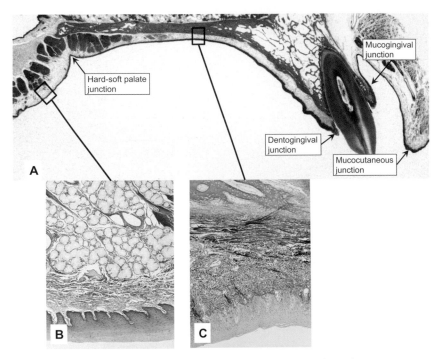

**Figure 6.1**   Junctions in the oral mucosa. (A) Histologic section cut sagittally through the mandible and anterior vestibule showing the junction between the lining mucosa (enlarged in B) of the soft palate and the masticatory mucosa of the hard palate (enlarged in C), the interface between the masticatory mucosa of the gingiva and the enamel of the tooth (dentogingival junction), the interface between the attached gingiva and the alveolar mucosa (mucogingival junction), and the interface between the skin and the oral mucosa (mucocutaneous junction).

more detailed description follows below. Finally, a brief account is given of junctions between different types of mucosa that are of morphologic interest and clinical importance (Fig. 6.1A).

## 6.1.1 Masticatory mucosa

Masticatory mucosa covers those areas of the oral cavity such as the hard palate and gingiva (Fig. 6.1A) that are exposed to compressive and shear forces and to abrasion during the mastication of food (see Fig. 2.1). The dorsum of the tongue has the same functional role as other masticatory mucosa but, because of its specialized structure, it is considered separately.

The epithelium of masticatory mucosa is moderately thick. It is frequently orthokeratinized, although normally there are parakeratinized areas of the gingiva and occasionally of the palate. Both types of epithelial surface are inextensible and are well adapted to withstanding abrasion. The junction between epithelium and underlying lamina propria is convoluted, and the numerous elongated papillae probably provide good mechanical attachment and prevent the epithelium from being stripped off under shear force. The lamina propria is thick, containing a dense network of collagen fibers in the form of large, closely packed bundles (Fig. 6.1C). They follow a direct course between anchoring points so that there is relatively little slack and the tissue does not yield on impact, enabling the mucosa to resist heavy loading.

Masticatory mucosa covers immobile structures (e.g., the hard palate and alveolar processes) and is firmly bound to them either directly by the attachment of lamina propria to the periosteum of underlying bone—such as in mucoperiosteum— or indirectly by a fibrous submucosa. In the lateral regions of the hard palate, this fibrous submucosa is interspersed with areas of fat and glandular tissue that cushion the mucosa against mechanical loads and protect the underlying nerves and blood vessels of the palate.

As already mentioned in Chapter 2, the firmness of masticatory mucosa ensures that it does not gape after surgical incisions (see Fig. 2.4B) and rarely requires suturing. For the same reason, injections of local anesthetic into these areas are difficult and are often painful, as is any swelling arising from inflammation.

## 6.1.2 Lining mucosa

The oral mucosa covering the underside of the tongue, inside of the lips, cheeks, floor of the mouth, and alveolar processes as far as the gingiva is mobile. These regions, together with the soft palate, are classified as lining mucosa (see Fig. 2.1).

The epithelium of lining mucosa is thicker than that of masticatory mucosa, sometimes exceeding 500 µm in the cheek, and is non-keratinized. The surface is thus flexible and is able to withstand stretching. The interface with connective tissue is relatively smooth, although slender connective tissue papillae often penetrate into the epithelium.

The lamina propria is generally thicker than in masticatory mucosa and contains fewer collagen fibers, which follow a more irregular course between anchoring points (Fig. 6.1B). Thus, the mucosa can be stretched to a certain extent before these fibers become taut and limit further distention. Associated with the collagen fibers are elastic fibers that tend to control the extensibility of the mucosa. Where lining mucosa covers muscle, it is attached by a mixture of collagen and elastic fibers. As the mucosa becomes slack during masticatory movements, the elastic fibers retract the mucosa toward the muscle and so prevent it from bulging between the teeth and being bitten.

The alveolar mucosa and the floor of the mouth mucosa are loosely attached to the underlying structures by a thick submucosa. In contrast, mucosa of the underside of the tongue is firmly bound to the underlying muscle. The soft palate is flexible but not highly mobile, and its mucosa is separated from the loose and highly glandular submucosa by a layer of elastic fibers.

The tendency for lining mucosa to be flexible, with a loose and often elastic submucosa, means that surgical incisions frequently require sutures for closure (see Fig. 2.4A). Injections into such regions are easy because there is ready dispersion of fluid in the loose connective tissue; however, infections also spread rapidly. The lining mucosa of the floor of the mouth and underside of tongue is thinner and is more permeable than the other regions (see Chapter 8) and, consequently, has been used for systemic delivery of pharmaceutical agents and local delivery of antigens to elicit mucosal immune response.

## 6.1.3 Specialized mucosa

The mucosa of the dorsal surface of the tongue is unlike that anywhere else in the oral cavity because, although covered by what is functionally a masticatory mucosa, it is also a highly extensible lining and, in addition, has different types of lingual papillae. Some of them possess a mechanical function, whereas others bear taste buds and therefore have a sensory function.

The mucous membrane of the tongue is composed of two parts, with different embryologic origins, and is divided by the V-shaped groove, the sulcus terminalis (terminal groove). The anterior two-thirds of the tongue, where the mucosa is derived from the first pharyngeal arch, is often called the *body*, and the posterior third, where the mucosa is derived from the third pharyngeal arch, the *base*. The mucosa covering the base of the tongue contains extensive nodules of lymphoid tissue, the lingual tonsils.

### Fungiform papillae

The anterior portion of the tongue bears the *fungiform* ("funguslike") and *filiform* ("hairlike") papillae (Fig. 6.2A). Single fungiform papillae are scattered between the numerous filiform papillae at the tip of the tongue (Fig. 6.2B). They are smooth, round structures that appear red because of their highly vascular connective tissue core, visible through a thin, non-keratinized covering epithelium. Taste buds are normally present in the epithelium on the superior surface.

### Filiform papillae

Filiform papillae cover the entire anterior part of the tongue and consist of cone-shaped structures, each with a core of connective tissue, covered by a thick keratinized epithelium (Fig. 6.2C). Together, they form a tough, abrasive surface that is involved in compressing and breaking food when the tongue is apposed to the hard palate. Thus, the dorsal mucosa of the tongue functions as a masticatory mucosa. Buildup of keratin results in elongation of the filiform

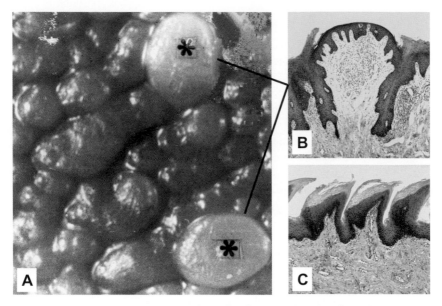

**Figure 6.2** Lingual papillae from the dorsal surface of the tongue. (A) Fungiform papillae are interspersed among numerous filiform papillae on the anterior of the tongue, two of which are evident (asterisks). (B,C) Histologic sections of the papillae in (A) show that the epithelium of the fungiform papilla is thinly keratinized or non-keratinized (B) and that of the filiform papillae is keratinized (C).

papillae in some patients. The dorsum of the tongue then has a "hairy" appearance called *hairy tongue.*

The tongue is highly extensible, with changes in its shape accommodated by the regions of non-keratinized, flexible epithelium between the filiform papillae.

### Foliate papillae

*Foliate* ("leaflike") papillae are sometimes present on the lateral margins of the posterior part of the tongue, although they are more frequently seen in mammals other than humans (Fig. 6.3A). These pink-colored papillae consist of 4– 11 parallel ridges that alternate with deep grooves in the mucosa, and numerous taste buds are present in the epithelium of the lateral walls of the ridges (Fig. 6.3B).

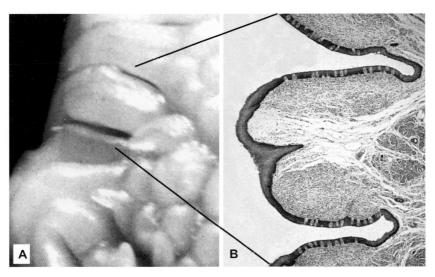

**Figure 6.3** (A) Ridge-shaped foliate papillae are another type of lingual papillae located laterally on the tongue. (B) A histological section through the area marked in (A) shows the epithelium covering the papillae is non-keratinized; the borders of the papillae are represented as deep grooves in the mucosa.

### Circumvallate papillae

Adjacent and anterior to the sulcus terminalis are 8–12 *circumvallate* ("walled") papillae, large structures each surrounded by a deep, circular groove into which open the ducts of minor salivary glands (the glands of von Ebner) (Fig. 6.4). These papillae have a connective tissue core that is covered on the superior surface by a keratinized epithelium. The epithelium covering the lateral walls is non-keratinized and contains numerous taste buds (Fig. 6.4B).

# 6.2 JUNCTIONS IN THE ORAL MUCOSA

## 6.2.1 Mucocutaneous junction

The skin, which contains hair follicles and sebaceous and sweat glands, is continuous with the oral mucosa at the lips (Figs. 6.1 and 6.5). Here, there is a transitional region where

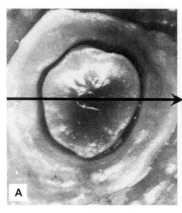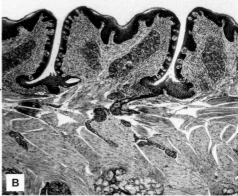

**Figure 6.4**  The circumvallate papillae (A) are situated in a row anterior to the sulcus terminalis on the dorsal surface of the tongue. (B) A histologic section through the papilla shows the superior surface of the papilla is covered by epithelium with a thin keratinized layer; that of the lateral walls is non-keratinized and contains many taste buds. Ducts of minor salivary glands open between the papillae.

appendages are absent except for a few sebaceous glands (situated mainly at the angles of the mouth). The epithelium of this region is keratinized but thin, with long connective tissue papillae containing capillary loops. This arrangement brings the blood close to the surface and accounts for the strong red coloration in this region, called the *red* (or *vermilion*) *zone* of the lip. The line separating the vermilion zone from the hair-bearing skin of the lip is called the *vermilion border*. In young persons, this border is sharply demarcated, but as a person is exposed to ultraviolet radiation, the border becomes diffuse and poorly defined.

Because the vermilion zone lacks salivary glands and contains few sebaceous glands, it tends to dry out, often becoming cracked and sore in cold weather. Between it and the thicker, non-keratinized labial mucosa is an intermediate zone covered by parakeratinized oral epithelium; studies of cytokeratins in this region show that K1 and K10, which are present in the epidermis and vermilion zone and associated with keratinization, are diminished. Conversely, there is also

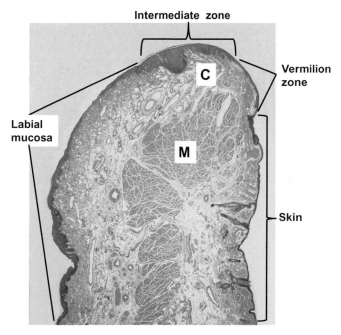

**Figure 6.5**    Sagittal section through the lip. The skin covering the external aspect has a thin epidermis and contains hair follicles. Continuous with this is the vermilion zone, which has a thin epithelium overlying an area of extensive vascularity containing numerous capillary loops (C). Between the vermilion zone and the labial mucosa of the oral cavity is the intermediate zone with a much thicker epithelium. There are minor salivary glands beneath the labial mucosa, and the extensive muscular tissue (M) represents part of the orbicularis oris.

a loss of K4 and K13 in this region, which are associated with non-keratinization (Barrett et al., 2005). In infants, the intermediate region is thickened and appears opalescent, which represents an adaptation to suckling, called the *suckling pad*.

## 6.2.2 Mucogingival junction

Although masticatory mucosa meets lining mucosa at several sites, none is more abrupt than the junction between attached gingiva and alveolar mucosa. This junction is identified clinically by a slight indentation called the *muco-gingival groove* and by the change from the bright pink of the alveolar mucosa to the paler pink of the gingiva (see Fig. 2.2A).

Histologically, there is a change at this junction, not only in the type of epithelium but also in the composition of the lamina propria (Fig. 6.1a and 6.6). The epithelium of the attached gingiva is keratinized or parakeratinized, and the lamina propria contains numerous coarse collagen bundles attaching the tissue to periosteum (Fig. 6.6B). The stippling seen clinically at the surface of healthy attached gingiva probably reflects the presence of this collagen attachment. The structure of mucosa changes at the mucogingival junction, where the alveolar mucosa has a thicker, non-keratinized epithelium overlying a loose lamina propria with numerous elastic fibers extending into the thick sub-mucosa (Fig. 6.6C). These elastic fibers return the alveolar mucosa to its original position after it is distended by the labial muscles during mastication and speech.

Coronal to the mucogingival junction is another clinically visible depression in the gingiva, the free gingival groove, whose level corresponds approximately to that of the bottom of the gingival sulcus (Fig. 6.6A). This demarcates the free and attached gingivae, although, unlike the mucogingival junction, there is no significant change in the structure of the mucosa at the free gingival groove.

### 6.2.3 The dentogingival junction

The region where the oral mucosa meets the surface of the tooth is a unique junction that is of considerable importance as it represents a potential weakness in the otherwise continuous epithelial lining of the oral cavity. The bacteria that are inevitably present on the tooth surface continually produce toxins capable of eliciting inflammation and damage if they enter the mucosal tissues. It is the junction between the epithelium and the enamel (Fig. 6.7) that is the principal seal between the oral cavity and the underlying tissues, and

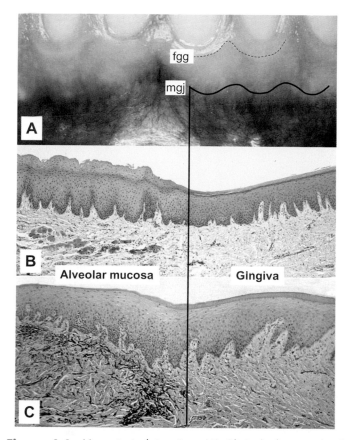

**Figure 6.6** Mucogingival junction. (A) Clinical photograph of healthy oral mucosa showing the mucogingival junction (mgj) evident as the interface between the pale pink of the attached gingiva and bright pink of the alveolar mucosa (solid wavy line). The boundary between the free and attached gingivae is demarcated by the free gingival groove (fgg), the level of which corresponds approximately to the bottom of the gingival sulcus (dashed line). (B,C) Histologic sections through the mucogingival junction (solid line). In (A) the differences in thickness, ridge pattern, and keratinization between epithelium of the gingiva and alveolar mucosa are seen; the section was stained by Papanicolaou's method, which reveals variations in keratinization. The junction in (B) was stained by Hart's method to demonstrate elastic fibers in the connective tissue. Although there is very little change in the epithelium in this specimen, a striking difference appears in the concentration of elastic fibers in the lamina propria between the masticatory gingiva and lining alveolar mucosa.

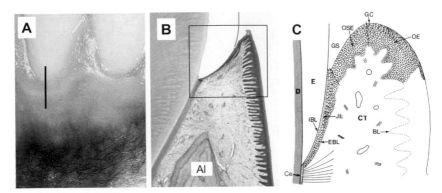

**Figure 6.7** (A) Clinical photograph of a healthy dentogingival junction, which represents the interface between the oral epithelium and the enamel of the tooth. (B) Histologic section of the dentogingival junction at the level indicated by the bar in (A). (Al, alveolar bone). (C) Diagram of the different types of epithelium from the outlined area of (B); oral (gingival) epithelium (OE); oral sulcular epithelium (OSE) and junctional epithelium (JE). The junctional epithelium is attached to the enamel of the tooth (E) by the internal basal lamina (IBL). Fibers of the periodontal ligament (deep connective tissue) insert into the cementum (Ce) of the tooth; BL, basal lamina of the gingival; CT, connective tissue; D, dentin; GC, gingival crest; GS, gingival sulcus; EBL, external basal lamina.

it is important to have an understanding of the nature of this union.

In the average human mouth, in which mild gingival inflammation is invariably present, the *gingival sulcus* (Fig. 6.7C, GS) has a depth of 0.5–3 mm, with an average of 1.8 mm. Any depth greater than 3 mm can generally be considered pathologic; a sulcus this deep is known as a periodontal pocket. When the tooth first becomes functional, the bottom of the sulcus is usually found on the cervical half of the anatomic crown; with age there is a gradual migration of the sulcus bottom, which eventually may pass on to the cementum surface. The sulcus contains fluid that has passed through the junctional epithelium and contains a mixture of both desquamated epithelial cells from the junctional and sulcular epithelia and polymorphonuclear leukocytes that have also passed through the junctional epithelium.

The floor of the sulcus and the epithelium cervical to it, which is applied to the tooth surface, is termed *junctional epithelium* (Fig. 6.7C, JE). The walls of the sulcus are lined by epithelium derived from, and continuous with, that of the rest of the oral mucosa. This has been designated *oral sulcular epithelium* (Fig. 6.7C, OSE) and has the same basic structure as non-keratinized oral epithelium elsewhere in the oral cavity. The ortho- or parakeratinized surface of the free gingiva (or oral epithelium, OE, Fig. 6.7C) is continuous with the oral sulcular epithelium at the level of the gingival crest (Fig. 6.7C, GC).

Junctional epithelium is derived from the reduced enamel (or dental) epithelium of the tooth germ. As the tooth erupts and the crown penetrates the overlying oral epithelium, there is fusion between the reduced enamel epithelium and the oral epithelium so that epithelial continuity is never lost. Morphologically, the junctional epithelium consists of flattened cells aligned parallel to the tooth surface and tapering from 3–4 layers in thickness apically to 15–30 layers coronally. The epithelium has a smooth connective tissue interface where there is an internal basal lamina (Fig. 6.8A,B) with associated hemidesmosomes and similar to that which attaches epithelium to connective tissue elsewhere in the oral mucosa. Between the plasma membrane of the junctional epithelial cells and the enamel (or, sometimes, cementum) surface, a basal lamina structure is present, associated with hemidesmosomes on the membranes of the epithelial cells (Fig. 6.8C). However, biochemical analysis has shown that although this basal lamina contains collagen VIII, it lacks other collagens found in normal basal laminae (type IV and type VII; see Table 5.2) and some of the proteoglycans; the laminin is also of a different type, known as laminin-5, rather than laminin-1 (Kinumatsu et al., 2008). The hemidesmosomes contain laminin-5 and integrin $\alpha6\beta4$ that interact with the basal lamina matrix. The junctional epithelial cells directly attached to the enamel have been termed DAT cells (Directly Attached to the Tooth; Pollanen et al., 2003).

The junctional epithelium is not simply an area of non-keratinized oral epithelium but a unique and poorly

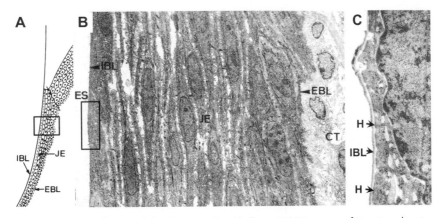

**Figure 6.8** Junctional epithelium. (A) Diagram of junctional epio-thelium (JE) showing the internal basal lamina (IBL) and external basal lamina (EBL). (B) Electron micrograph of the outlined area in (A) showing the attachment of the IBL to the enamel surface (ES) of the tooth. Note the lack of differentiation of the junctional epithelium and the wide intercellular spaces (CT, connective tissue). (C) Electron micrograph of the outlined area in (B) showing the fine structure of the attachment of a junctional epithelial cell to the enamel surface. Hemidesmosomes (H) are evident at the surface of the cell. ((B) from Schroeder and Listgarten, 1977. Reprinted with permission from S. Karger AG, Busel; (C) from Squier and Finkelstein, 2003, Copyright Mosby.)

differentiated tissue. Thus, the ultrastructural characteristics of junctional epithelial cells are relatively constant through-out the tissue and differ considerably from those of other oral epithelial cells. The amount of rough endoplasmic retic-ulum and Golgi complexes is significantly greater, as is the amount of cytoplasm. Conversely, far fewer tonofilaments and desmosomal junctions are present so it is resistant to mechanical stress than other regions of oral epithelium. The cytokeratins present represent those seen in basal epithelial cells (K5, K14, and K19) and in simple epithelia (K8, K18). Although junctional epithelium cells divide and migrate to the surface, they show no sign of differentiation to form a keratinized surface epithelium, and the small lipid-containing granules (*membrane-coating* or *lamellate* granules, associated with intercellular barrier formation) are absent. These features, as well as the frequent presence of polymorphonuclear leukocytes and mononuclear cells, may all contribute to the permeability of the tissue. This has been extensively studied and a variety of substances ranging from cells to tissue fluid and small protein molecules have been shown to be capable of traversing the epithelium. This makes the structure of the sulcus an important factor in the etiology and pathogenesis of periodontal disease.

As in all epithelia, the deeper cells adjacent to the connective tissue undergo cell division to replenish those lost at the surface. However, DAT cells are also capable of division and migrate coronally, parallel to the tooth surface, to be desquamated into the gingival sulcus (Pollanen et al., 2003).

One of the remarkable properties of the junctional epithelium is that it readily regenerates from the adjacent oral sulcular or oral epithelium if it is damaged or surgically excised (Bosshardt and Lang, 2005). The new junctional epithelium has all the characteristics of the original tissue, including the same types of cytokeratins and an attachment to the tooth that is indistinguishable from the original one. This raises interesting questions as to the nature of the inductive signals responsible for inducing the formation of this tissue. The best suggestion is that of a connective tissue influence, which is described later.

## The connective tissue component

As elsewhere in the oral mucosa, the lamina propria is divided into papillary and reticular components and contains collagen fibers, ground substance, cells, blood vessels, lymphatic vessels, and nerves.

## Blood supply

The lamina propria is heavily vascularized (Schroeder and Listgarten, 1997). It contains a vast network of postcapillary venules called the gingival plexus that encircles the tooth and extends from the coronal to the apical termination of the junctional epithelium. The blood supply to the gingiva is derived from periosteal vessels in the periosteum of the alveolar process. Branches from these vessels are perpendicular to the surface and form loops within the connective tissue papillae of the gingiva. Vessels supplying the dentogingival junction are derived from the continuation of interalveolar arteries as they pierce the alveolar crest. These vessels run parallel to the sulcular epithelium and form a rich network just below the basement membrane.

For descriptive purposes, the blood supply to the periodontium can be divided into three zones: (1) that to the periodontal ligament (PDL); (2) that to the gingiva facing the oral cavity; and (3) that to the gingiva facing the tooth. Connections among the three permit collateral circulation.

## Nerve supply

The gingival component of the periodontium is innervated by terminal branches of periodontal nerve fibers and by branches of the infraorbital and palatine, or lingual, mental, and buccal nerves. In the attached gingiva, most nerves terminate within the lamina propria, and only a few endings occur between epithelial cells. In the dentogingival junction of rat molars, a rich innervation of the junctional epithelium has been demonstrated, with free nerve endings between epithelial cells at both the connective tissue and the tooth surface of the epithelium. Vesicular structures and neuropeptides have been demonstrated in these nerve endings. Substance P-immunoreactive nerve bundles are present in the lamina propria beneath the junctional epithelium. Some nerve trunks produce branches in and near the basal layer of the apical two-thirds of the junctional epithelium. Although the exact biological significance of these nerves are not known, they may have a role in local tissue defense. Substance P released from neurons likely binds to neurokinin-1 receptors on junctional epithelial cells, endothelial cells, polymorphonuclear leukocytes, and monocytes. It also induces infiltration of polymorphonuclear leukocytes from blood vessels into the junctional epithelium and underlying connective tissue, induces cytokine production by monocytes, and increases permeability of blood vessels beneath the junctional epithelium.

## The col

Interdental gingiva appears to have the outline of a col (or depression), with buccal and lingual peaks guarding it. Col epithelium is identical to junctional epithelium, has the same origin (from dental epithelium), and is gradually replaced by continuing cell division. There is no evidence that the structural elements of the col increase vulnerability to periodontal disease. Rather, the incidence of gingivitis interdentally is greater than in other areas because the contours between the teeth allow bacteria, food debris, and plaque to accumulate in this location.

## The periodontal ligament

The PDL serves to link the teeth to the alveolar bone providing support and protection (Beertsen et al., 1997). This ligament is a unique and multifunctional connective tissue interposed between the cementum of the tooth root and the alveolar socket wall. It is derived from dental follicle and contains collagen, fibroblasts, epithelial rests of Malassez, and cementoblasts.

The PDL possesses the ability to regenerate lost connective tissue (Coura et al., 2008). This is thought to be due to the presence of PDL stem cells described as neural crest stem cells and mesenchymal stem cells that appear to be the precursors of fibroblasts, osteoblasts, and cementoblasts. When isolated from PDL, cells produce the markers nestin (neural stem cells) and HNK1 and p75 (undifferentiated neural crest cells), and STRO-1, CD44, and CD146 (mesenchymal stem cells). After growth-induced neural differentiation, neural stem cells express markers for β-tubulin III, neurofilament M, peripherin, microtubule-associated protein 2 and protein zero (Coura et al., 2008).

The PDL cells are also responsive to periodontal bacteria and express mRNA for IL-1β, IL-6, IL-8, TNF-α, RANKL, and osteoprotegerin after stimulation organisms. This suggests that these cells may play a role in cytokine production in periodontal disease (Krajewski et al., 2009).

## Inflammation in the dentogingival region

Examination of the connective tissue supporting epithelium of the dentogingival junction shows it to be structurally different from connective tissue supporting the oral gingival epithelium in that, even in clinically normal gingiva, it contains an inflammatory infiltrate thought to be initiated at the time of tooth eruption. Cells of the inflammatory series, particularly polymorphonuclear leukocytes, continually migrate into the junctional epithelium and pass between the epithelial cells to appear in the gingival sulcus and eventually in the oral fluid.

The cellular infiltrate in the lamina propria connective tissue is estimated to occupy 3%–6% of the gingival volume (Schroeder and Listgarten, 1997). The majority of these cells accumulate around the vessels and postcapillary venules in the gingival plexus in this area. The majority of these cells are T lymphocytes with lesser amounts of macrophages, B lymphocytes, plasma cells, and dendritic Langerhans cells.

The infiltrate in the connective tissue provides functional protection against infection. Microorganisms and microbial by-products pass through the highly permeable junctional epithelium and enter the lamina propria. These microbial antigens attract polymorphonuclear leukocytes and antigen presenting cells directly. They also stimulate local venules to express ELAM-1, ICAM-1, LFA-3, and VCAM-1 that attracts T cells via by their selectin and integrin surface receptors. Here, macrophages and Langerhans cells can present antigens to the T lymphocytes (Schroeder and Listgarten, 1997).

## Connective tissue and epithelial differentiation at the dentogingival junction

There is evidence that the connective tissue supporting junctional epithelium is functionally different from the connective tissue supporting the rest of the oral epithelium, and such a difference has important connotations for the pathogenesis of periodontal disease and regeneration of the dentogingival junction after periodontal surgery.

Tissue recombination experiments have shown that connective tissue plays a key role in determining epithelial expression. It has been proposed that subepithelial connective tissues (the lamina propria) provide "instructive" influences for the normal maturation of a stratified squamous epithelium, and these influences are absent from deep connective tissue, which possesses only "permissive" factors required to maintain the epithelium in a poorly differentiated, or immature, state (Mackenzie and Hill, 1984). Thus, epithelium combined with deep connective tissue does not mature but instead persists in a state closely resembling that of junctional epithelium.

At the dentogingival junction, it is believed that gingival and sulcular epithelia (supported by an instructive connective tissue) are able to mature, whereas junctional epithelium (supported by a deep connective tissue, the PDL) remains undifferentiated. This difference in phenotypic expression is important because, by retaining a degree of immaturity, the junctional epithelium can develop hemidesmosomal attachments where its cells come into contact with the tooth surface.

It has already been stated that the connective tissue associated with the dentogingival junction is inflamed. This inflammation also influences epithelial expression. Thus, the oral sulcular epithelium, in marked distinction to the gingival epithelium, is non-keratinized, yet both are supported by gingival lamina propria. This difference in epithelial expression may be a direct consequence of the inflammatory process which may influence the production of keratinocyte growth factors (keratinocyte growth factor-1, Li et al., 2005). The junctional epithelium is also influenced by inflammation, and when inflammation increases, there is active proliferation and migration of the junctional epithelium, resulting in a periodontal pocket and apical movement of attachment level.

# REFERENCES

Barrett, A.W., Morgan, M., Nwaeze, G., Kramer, G., and Berkovitz, B.K. (2005) The differentiation profile of the epithelium of the human lip. Arch Oral Biol 50:431–438.

Beertsen, W., McCulloch, C.A., and Sodek, J. (1997) The periodontal ligament: a unique, multifunctional connective tissue. Periodontology 13:20–40.

Bosshardt, D.D., and Lang, N.P. (2005) The junctional epithelium: from health to disease. J Dent Res 84:9–20.

Coura, G.S., Garcez, R.C., de Aguiar, C.B., Alvarez-Silva, M., Magini, R.S., and Trentin, A.G. (2008) Human periodontal ligament: a niche of neural crest stem cells. J Periodontal Res 43:531–536.

Kinumatsu, T., Hashimoto, S., Muramatsu, T., Sasaki, H., Jung, H.S., Yamada, S., and Shimono, M. (2008) Involvement of laminin and integrins in adhesion and migration of junctional epithelium cells. J Periodontal Res 44:13–20.

Krajewski, A.C., Biessei, J., Kunze, M., Maersch, S., Perabo, L., and Noack, M.J. (2009) Influence of lipopolysaccharide and interleukin-6 on RANKL and OPG expression and release in human periodontal ligament cells. APMIS 117:746–754.

Li, M., Firth, J.D., and Putnins, E.E. (2005) Keratinocyte growth factor-1 expression in healthy and diseased human periodontal tissues. J Periodontal Res 40:118–128.

Mackenzie, I.C., and Hill, M.W. (1984) Connective tissue influences on patterns of epithelial architecture and keratinization in skin and oral mucosa of the adult mouse. Cell Tissue Res 235(3):551–559.

Pollanen, M.T., Salonen, J.I., and Uitto, V.J. (2003) Structure and function of the tooth-epithelial interface in health and disease. Periodontology 31:12–31.

Schroeder, H.E., and Listgarten, M.A. (1977) Fine structure of the developing epithelial attachment of human teeth. In: Monographs in Developmental Biology Vol. 2 (A. Wolsky, ed.) p. 47. S. Karger AG, Basel.

Schroeder, H.E., and Listgarten, M.A. (1997) The gingival tissues: the architecture of periodontal protection. Periodontology 13:91–120.

Squier, C.A., and Finkelstein, M.W. (2003) Oral mucosa. In: Ten Cate's Oral Histology, Development, Structure and Function (A. Nanci, ed.) pp. 329–375. Mosby, St. Louis, MO.

# Development and aging of the oral mucosa

Although all oral mucosa is composed of a stratified epithelium supported by connective tissue, there are marked regional differences that were described in the previous chapter. Minor variations may be superimposed on this basic pattern, such as keratinization of the buccal mucosa along the occlusal line, but the basic regional differences are predetermined and develop early in the embryo. As has been mentioned earlier, the type of epithelium that develops in a particular site appears to be determined primarily by the connective tissue on which it rests, both during embryonic development and in the adult, and instructions pass between these two components of the mucosa throughout the life of the tissue. These so-called epithelial-mesenchymal interactions are considered in more detail later, and first we briefly describe the developmental stages of oral mucosa.

*Human Oral Mucosa: Development, Structure, and Function.* Edited by Christopher Squier and Kim A. Brogden.
© 2011 Christopher Squier and Kim A. Brogden. Published 2011 by John Wiley & Sons, Inc.

# 7.1 DEVELOPMENTAL STAGES OF ORAL MUCOSA

The primitive oral cavity develops by fusion of the embryonic stomatodeum with the foregut after rupture of the buccopharyngeal membrane, at about 26 days of gestation, and thus comes to be lined by epithelium derived from both ectoderm and endoderm. The precise boundary between these two embryonic tissues is poorly defined, but structures that develop in the branchial arches (e.g., tongue, epiglottis, pharynx) are covered by epithelium derived from endoderm, whereas the epithelium covering the palate, cheeks, floor of mouth, gingivae, and lips is of ectodermal origin (Winning and Townsend, 2000).

By 5 to 6 weeks of gestation, the single layer of epithelial cells lining the primitive oral cavity has formed five or more layers, and by 8–10 weeks, there is a multilayered epithelium with marked thickening in the region of the vestibular dental lamina complex. In the central region of this thickening, cellular degeneration occurs at 10 to 14 weeks, resulting in separation of the cells covering the cheek area and the alveolar mucosa and thus forming the oral vestibule. At about this time (8–11 weeks), the palatal shelves elevate and close, so that the future morphology of the adult oral cavity is apparent.

At this stage, the future lamina propria is composed of a subectodermal condensation of branching cells with a minimal, intercellular fibrillar component. A denser fibrillar accumulation along the epithelial interface heralds the development of the basement membrane. All areas are now lined with multilayered ectoderm, and it becomes possible to distinguish sites destined for keratinization, such as the alveolar ridge and hard palate, from those that will be non-keratinized, like cheek, lip, and soft palate. The future keratinized regions have columnar basal cells, tonofilaments, and cytoplasmic processes projecting into the mesenchyme.

Between 7 and 10 weeks, the surface features of the oral mucosa such as the incisive papilla and palatal rugae are developing. The lingual epithelium shows specialization at about 7 weeks when the circumvallate and foliate papillae first appear, followed by the fungiform papillae. Within these papillae, taste buds soon develop. The filiform papillae that cover most of the anterior two-thirds of the tongue become apparent at about 10 weeks. By 10 to 12 weeks, the future lining and masticatory regions show stratification of the epithelium and different morphology. Those areas destined to become keratinized (e.g., hard palate and alveolar ridge of gingiva) have darkly staining, columnar basal cells that are separated from the underlying connective tissue by a prominent basement membrane. Short connective tissue papillae are also evident. By contrast, the epithelium that will form areas of lining mucosa retains cuboidal basal cells, and the epithelium–connective tissue interface remains relatively flat. In the mesenchyme, capillary buds and reticulin fibers appear, and in the future masticatory regions, there are more cells and fibers, including collagen, evident from weeks 8 to 11 (Winning and Townsend, 2000). Although the collagen initially shows no particular orientation, as the fibers increase in number, they tend to form bundles; immediately subjacent to the epithelium, these bundles are perpendicular to the basement membrane.

In skin, a distinctive surface layer known as a periderm develops at 8 weeks. It is composed of large, bulbous cells which give the surface an undulating appearance and which are shed into the amniotic cavity. This layer is retained until a keratinized layer has differentiated beneath it by week 26, after which it is shed. Although the term periderm has been used to describe the surface layer of developing oral epithelium, it is never as distinctive as that on the embryonic skin surface, although it may be seen in the region of the mucocutaneous junction (see Fig. 7.1B).

Between 13 and 20 weeks of gestation, the oral epithelia thicken, reaching 15 cell layers in some regions (Fig. 7.1). Desmosomes are well formed, and the "prickle cell" character of the mid-level cells is apparent while the development of sparse keratohyalin granules permits a distinction between the prickle cells and granular layer. At the end of this period (20–24 weeks), the surface layers of masticatory

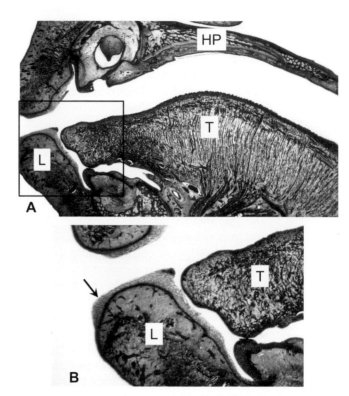

**Figure 7.1** (A) Part of a sagittal section through the oral cavity of a 15-week human embryo showing the tongue (T), floor of the mouth, alveolar ridge with a tooth bud *in situ*, hard palate (HP), and lip (L). Differences in thickness are already apparent between the epithelia of the labial mucosa, alveolar ridge, floor of the mouth, and tongue, and papillae are evident on the dorsum of the tongue. (B) Enlargement of the outlined area in (A) showing the distinctive surface layer of periderm (*arrow*) on the lip.

mucosa appear parakeratinized; orthokeratin is not thought to be present until after the teeth erupt during the postnatal period, at approximately 6 months after birth. Cytokeratins, a marker of epithelial differentiation, are similar in all mucosal regions until 10 weeks and resemble those of the adult lining epithelium, with the addition of cytokeratins 8, 18, and 19 (Pelissier et al., 1992). From week 11, regions of masticatory mucosa (gingiva and hard palate) begin to develop cytokeratins characteristic of these sites (cytokeratins 1, 2, 10, and 11). Involucrin can be detected at 9 weeks and reaches levels found in adult tissue by 15 weeks (Klein-Szanto, 1985).

In the lamina propria, the network of mesenchymal cells lose contact with their neighbors and are recognizable as fibroblasts. Collagen fibers increase in number and size, and between 16 and 20 weeks, the elastic fibers become prominent in the future regions of lining mucosa. The basement membrane becomes more clearly defined and hemidesmosomes and basal lamina anchoring fibrils appear. Epithelial ridges elongate in future masticatory regions.

Melanoblasts, the precursors of melanocytes, arise from neural crest cells and migrate into the oral mucosa from the 11th week onward. Once in the epithelium, melanocytes form a self-perpetuating population for which the microphthalmia transcription factor, MITF, appears to be important for proliferation and maintenance (Lin and Fisher, 2007). Langerhans cells appear in oral mucosa at the same time as melanocytes and are probably capable of division so as to maintain a local population, although circulating precursors may augment these cells in damaged tissue (Barrett et al., 1996).

Merkel cells have been detected in oral epithelium at the 16th week of gestation and have been claimed to have a neural crest origin like melanoblasts. However, their lack of similarity to melanocytes and their resemblance to keratinocytes in terms of the presence of desmosomes and cytokeratin suggest that they may represent modified keratinocytes and arise from division of these cells (Lucarz and Brand, 2007).

Minor salivary gland primordia appear at the 8th week and grow as solid branching cords of epithelium which later develop a lumen and thus form ducts. The secretory portion forms later around the ends of the finer ducts.

## 7.2 THE CONTROL OF MUCOSAL DEVELOPMENT: EPITHELIAL–MESENCHYMAL INTERACTION

It is reasonable to assume that cells derived from the fertilized ovum initially possess the same genetic information but that during differentiation to form cells with different structure and function, there is a progressive restriction of this information so only information necessary for a particular pathway of differentiation is available. At this stage, a cell can be said to be *determined*, determination representing the final step in a series of restrictive changes.

The process of differentiation is thought to be brought about by an inductive mechanism, and there are many experiments which suggest that the mesenchyme exerts a dominant controlling or inductive influence on epithelial differentiation (reviewed by Rinn et al., 2008). If the dermal component of embryonic skin is separated from the ectoderm, the ectoderm not only fails to differentiate but eventually dies. If recombined with its own mesenchyme, then normal differentiation follows.

As all covering and lining epithelia are continuously renewing cell populations, the question arises as to whether this control continues to be exercised in subsequent generations of cells and eventually in adult tissues. Recent work on tissue-specific stem cells in animal models suggest that control does continue to be exercised in tissues leading to subsequent generations of cells (see e.g., Bertrand et al., 2010). In the oral cavity, experimental evidence based on recombination and transplantation of dermal and epidermal components from various sites suggests that the dermis does appear to control the type of epidermis growing at the graft site (Mackenzie and Hill, 1984). This fact is of relevance to surgical procedures; for example, if skin is grafted into the mouth to replace an area of excised mucosa, it retains all the characteristics of the donor site including hairs, because the dermis invariably forms part of the thickness of the graft. Likewise, in periodontal surgical procedures, where flaps of oral mucosa are repositioned about the necks of teeth, the

donor site determines the characteristics of the newly posi-
tioned tissue: non-keratinized alveolar mucosa advanced to
the gingival will not take on the characteristics of the keratinized gingival mucosa in spite of altered functional
demands at this site.

However, not all experiments have provided such clear-
cut evidence, For example, when epithelia from hamster
tongue, palate, and cheek pouch were combined with
footpad epidermis, the epithelial specificity was retained.
Trunk epidermis, on the other hand, was able to induce
tongue epithelium to form epidermis. These and other
experiments suggest there may be a degree of reciprocity
between the epithelium and connective tissue in the determination of epithelial character by the mesoderm (Rinn
et al., 2008). There is considerable evidence that fibroblasts
in the mesenchyme produce the primary signals that determines the fate of the overlying epithelium. Fibroblasts are a
diverse population and are highly site-specific in terms of
gene expression associated with extracellular matrix synthesis, lipid metabolism, and signaling pathways controlling
cell migration and cell differentiation (Chang et al., 2002). A
factor produced by fibroblasts, keratinocyte growth factor
(KGF, also known as KGF-1 or fibroblast growth factor-7)
stimulates epithelia proliferation (Werner et al., 2007). The
reciprocity between epithelial keratinocytes and connective
tissue fibroblasts has given rise to the concept of "double
paracrine signaling" by which keratinocytes may initiate
production of growth factors in fibroblasts which in turn
stimulate keratinocyte proliferation (Werner et al., 2007). The
keratinocyte-derived factors that can stimulate both the
keratinocytes themselves and fibroblasts and other mes-
enchmal cell types include TGF-β, platelet-derived growth
factor (PDGF), and IL-1. The effects of these factors are inter-
related; TGF-β induces expression of IL-1 and both TGF-β
and IL-1 induce expression of PDGF. TGF-β is a potent
growth inhibitor for keratinocytes and fibroblasts at lower
concentrations yet promotes proliferation of these cells at
higher concentrations. PDGF is a chemoattractant for fibroblasts, and IL-1, among its many properties, stimulates proliferation and activation of fibroblasts.

Although KGF-1 is typically expressed by connective tissue cells and acts on epithelium to maintain tissue stability, it may be produced by gingival epithelium and upregulated in inflamed tissue, thereby contributing to increased proliferation and formation of pocket epithelium, as mentioned in Chapter 6 (Li et al., 2005).

## 7.3 AGING

Aging has been defined as the slow, inexorable, cumulative changes which occur with chronological age and which limit the ability of the organism to respond to the challenge of disease or the environment. Such changes are more evident in skin than in mucosa.

Clinically, the oral mucosa of an elderly person often has a smoother, glossy, and dryer surface than that of a young person and may be described as atrophic or friable (Fig. 7.2), but it is likely that these changes represent the cumulative effects of systemic disease, drug therapy, or both, rather than an intrinsic biologic aging process of the mucosa.

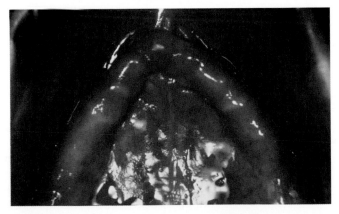

**Figure 7.2** Clinical photograph of the edentulous maxilla of an elderly person. The oral mucosa appears smooth and shiny. (Illustration courtesy of Dr. R.L. Ettinger.)

Histologically, the epithelium appears thinner, and a smoothing of the epithelium–connective tissue interface results from the flattening of epithelial ridges; these changes are usually most evident in lip, cheek, and lateral border of tongue. There is a decrease in the number of cells in the connective tissue (Cruchley and Williams, 1994) with an increased amount of collagen, which is believed to become more highly cross-linked. Sebaceous glands (Fordyce's spots) of the lips and cheeks also increase with age, and the minor salivary glands show marked atrophy with fibrous replacement.

The dorsum of the tongue may show a reduction in the number of filiform papillae and a smooth or glossy appearance, such changes being exacerbated by any nutritional deficiency of iron or B complex vitamins. The reduced number of filiform papillae may make the fungiform papillae more prominent, and patients may erroneously consider it to be a disease state.

Aging is associated with decreased rates of metabolic activity, and studies on epidermis show a tendency for epithelial proliferation and rate of tissue turnover to decrease with age. However, in healthy oral tissue, there is no good evidence for change in these parameters with age in humans or animals (Hill, 1994).

Langerhans cells decrease in skin in animals and possibly, in humans (Czernielewski et al., 1988; Thiers et al., 1984) but not in oral mucosa (Farthing and Walton, 1994). Nevertheless, cell-mediated immunity decreases with age (Weksler, 1982), and there is decreased cytokine production (Sauder et al., 1989).

## 7.3.1 Effect of age on wound healing

A delay in epithelial migration and proliferation has been described in wounds in mouse skin and mucosa, but there is no overall impairment of healing (Hill et al., 1994). In a study of healing after periodontal surgery in 80 patients, there were no differences attributable to age providing there was impeccable oral hygiene (Lindhe et al., 1985).

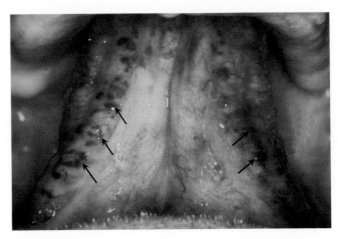

**Figure 7.3** Clinical photograph of ventral surface of the tongue in an elderly person showing varicosities (*arrows*). (Illustration courtesy of Dr. R.L. Ettinger, reprinted from Squier and Finkelstein, 2003, Copyright Mosby.)

## 7.3.2 Effect of aging on the vascular system and blood flow

Vascular changes may be quite prominent, with the development of varicosities (Fig. 7.3), sometimes called *caviar tongue* on the undersurface of the tongue (Ettinger and Manderson, 1974). Although such changes appear to be unrelated to the cardiovascular status of the patient, they are more frequent in patients with varicose veins of the legs. Functionally, there is no evidence for changes in blood flow in human oral mucosa in the absence of disease but reduced blood flow has been described in palate and dorsal tongue in aged rats (Hill et al., 1987).

## 7.3.3 Aging and the oral environment

Elderly patients, particularly postmenopausal women, may present with symptoms such as dryness of the mouth, burning sensations, and abnormal taste, but longitudinal studies suggest that there is no decrease in salivary flow rates with age in the absence of disease or medication (Baum, 1981; Tylenda et al., 1988). However, there is a decrease in the mucins (MG1 and MG2) that coat the mucosa and limit colonization by microorganisms (Denny et al., 1991), and many older individuals do have disease or are on medications that decrease salivary flow.

# REFERENCES

Barrett, A.W., Cruchley, A.T., and Williams, D.M. (1996) Oral mucosal Langerhans cells. Crit Rev Oral Biol Med 7(1):36–58.

Baum, B.J. (1981) Research on aging and oral health: an assessment of current status and future needs. Spec Care Dentist 1(4):156–165.

Bertrand, J.Y., Chi, C.C., Santoso, B., Teng, S., Stainier, D.Y., and Traver, D. (2010) Haematopoietic stem cells derive directly from aortic endothelium during development. Nature 464:108–111.

Chang, H.Y., Chi, J.-T., Dudoit, S., Bondre, C., van de Rijn, M., Botstein, D., and Brown, P.O. (2002) Diversity, topographic differentiation, and positional memory in human fibroblasts. Proc Natl Acad Sci U S A 99:12877–12882.

Cruchley, A.T., and Williams, D.M. (1994) Langerhans cell density in normal human oral mucosa and skin: relationship to age, smoking and alcohol consumption. J Oral Pathol Med 23(2):55–59.

Czernielewski, M., Masouye, I., Pisani, A., Ferracin, J., Auvolat, D., and Ortonne, J.P. (1988) Effect of chronic sun exposure on human Langerhans cell densities. Photodermatology 5:116–120.

Denny, P.C., Denny, P.A., Klauser, D.K., Hong, S.H., Navazesh, M., and Tabak, L.A. (1991) Age-related changes in mucins from human whole saliva. J Dent Res 70:1320–1327.

Ettinger, R.L., and Manderson, R.D. (1974) A clinical study of sublingual varices. Oral Surg Oral Med Oral Pathol 38:540–545.

Farthing, P.M., and Walton, L.J. (1994) Changes in immune function with age. In: The Effect of Aging in Oral Mucosa and

Skin (C.A. Squier and M.W. Hill, eds.) pp. 113–120. CRC Press, Boca Raton, FL.

Hill, M.W. (1994) Epithelial proliferation and turnover in oral epithelium and epidermis with age. In: The Effect of Aging in Oral Mucosa and Skin (C.A. Squier and M.W. Hill, eds.) pp. 75–83. CRC Press, Boca Raton, FL.

Hill, M.W., Squier, C.A., and Peston, P. (1987) Blood flow in skin and oral mucosa of young and old rats. J Dent Res 66(Special Issue):1053.

Hill, M.W., Karthigasan, J., Berg, J.H., and Squier, C.A. (1994) Influence of age on the response of oral mucosa to injury. In: The Effect of Aging in Oral Mucosa and Skin (C.A. Squier and M.W. Hill, eds.) pp. 129–142. CRC Press, Boca Raton, FL.

Klein-Szanto, A.J. (1985) Distribution of keratins and involucrin in human fetal oral epithelia. Acta Odontol Latinoam 2:35–41.

Li, M., Firth, J.D., and Putnins, E.E. (2005) Keratinocyte growth factor-1 expression in healthy and diseased human periodontal tissues. J Periodontal Res 40:118–128.

Lin, J.Y., and Fisher, D.E. (2007) Melanocyte biology and skin pigmentation. Nature 445(7130):843–850.

Lindhe, J., Socransky, S., Nyman, S., Westfelt, E., and Haffajee, A. (1985) Effect of aging on healing following periodontal therapy. J Clin Peridontol 12:774–787.

Lucarz, A., and Brand, G. (2007) Current considerations about Merkel cells. Eur J Cell Biol 86(5):243–251.

Mackenzie, I.C., and Hill, M.W. (1984) Connective tissue influences on patterns of epithelial architecture and keratinization in skin and oral mucosa of the adult mouse. Cell Tissue Res 235(3):551–559.

Pelissier, A., Ouhayoun, J.P., Sawaf, M.H., and Forest, N. (1992) Changes in cytokeratin expression during the development of the human oral mucosa. J Periodontal Res 27:588–598.

Rinn, J.L., Wang, J.K., Liu, H., Montgomery, K., van de Rijn, M., and Chang, H.Y. (2008) A systems biology approach to anatomic diversity of skin. J Invest Dermatol 128(4):776–782.

Sauder, D.N., Ponnappan, U., and Cinader, B. (1989) Effect of age on cutaneous interleukin 1 expression. Immunol Lett 20:111–114.

Squier, C.A., and Finkelstein, M.W. (2003) Oral mucosa. In: Ten Cate's Oral Histology, Development, Structure and Function (A. Nanci, ed.) pp. 329–375. Mosby, St. Louis, MO.

Thiers, B.H., Maize, J.C., Spicer, S.S., and Cantor, A.B. (1984) The effect of aging and chronic sun exposure on human Langerhans cell population. J Invest Dermatol 82:223–226.

Tylenda, C.A., Ship, J.A., and Baum, B.J. (1988) Evaluation of submandibular salivary flow rate in different age groups. J Dent Res 67(9):1225–1228.

Weksler, M.E. (1982) Age-associated changes in the immune response. J Am Geriatr Soc 30:718–723.

Werner, S., Krieg, T., and Smola, H. (2007) Keratinocyte-fibroblast interactions in wound healing. J Invest Derm 127:998–1008.

Winning, T.A., and Townsend, G.C. (2000) Oral mucosal embryology and histology. Clin Dermatol 18:499–511.

# Barrier functions of oral mucosa

The important function of the oral epithelium in protecting the underlying tissues and glands of the oral mucosa has already been mentioned in Chapter 1. This protective role includes the ability to resist mechanical damage resulting from activities such as mastication, to limit the entry of toxins and microorganisms present in the oral cavity, and to mount an immunoprotective response should they do so.

The patterns of differentiation in oral epithelium that produce a surface layer with appropriate properties to resist the forces to which it is subject have been described in detail in Chapter 3. These are principally *keratinization*, in which surface-cornified cells become filled with a compact array of condensed cytokeratin filaments, bounded by a thickened cell envelope and surrounded by an external lipid matrix, and *non-keratinization* in which the mature cells in the outer portion of the epithelium become large and flat and possess a cross-linked protein envelope, but retain nuclei and other organelles, and the cytokeratins do not aggregate to form

*Human Oral Mucosa: Development, Structure, and Function.* Edited by Christopher Squier and Kim A. Brogden.
© 2011 Christopher Squier and Kim A. Brogden. Published 2011 by John Wiley & Sons, Inc.

bundles of filaments as seen in keratinizing epithelia. This chapter will describe the characteristics of the permeability barrier and immunoprotective responses in oral mucosa.

# 8.1 THE PERMEABILITY BARRIER

As cells leave the basal layer and enter into differentiation, they become larger and begin to flatten and to accumulate lipids. A portion of the accumulating lipid is packaged in small organelles known as membrane-coating granules or lamellar granules that become evident in the prickle cell layer (see Fig. 8.1) (Martinez and Peters, 1971). At the boundary between the granular and cornified layers, the membrane-coating granules migrate to the superficial (apical) aspect of the keratinocyte, where the bounding membrane of the organelle fuses with the cell plasma membrane so that the lipid lamellae are extruded into the extracellular spaces of the surface layer (Landmann, 1988). Here it undergoes enzymatic processing to produce a lipid mixture consisting of ceramides, cholesterol, and fatty acids. This intercellular lipid is uniquely organized into a multilamellar complex that fills most of the intercellular space of the stratum corneum. The barrier properties of the stratum corneum are related to the phase behavior of the intercellular lipids. Thus, the membrane-coating granules are believed to be responsible for the formation of the superficial permeability barrier in stratified squamous epithelium; the evidence for this is presented in a subsequent section.

→

**Figure 8.1**  Diagram to show the major structural changes during maturation and formation of the permeability barrier in keratinized epithelium. Insert: Membrane-coating granules are formed in the Golgi region (gr) in the prickle cell layer and migrate to the superficial cell membrane as cells reach the granular layer. Here, the membrane of the granule (gcm) fuses with the cell plasma membrane, and the lipid lamellae (lb) are extruded into the intercellular space and become rearranged into intercellular lamellae (icl) that lie parallel to the horny cell envelope (hec) of the keratinized cell, containing keratin filaments (kf). We are grateful to Dr. Philip Wertz for providing the insert.

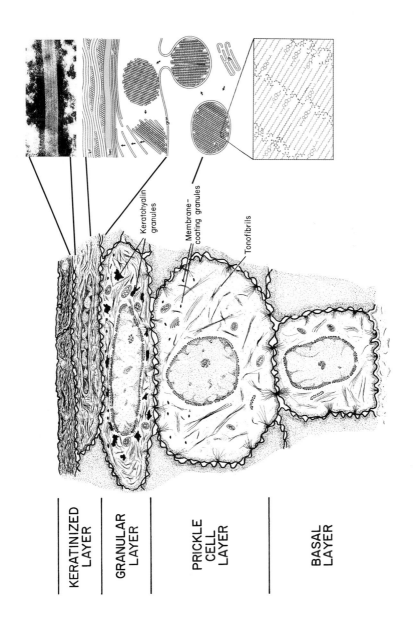

Keratohyalin granules

Membrane-coating granules

Tonofibrils

KERATINIZED LAYER

GRANULAR LAYER

PRICKLE CELL LAYER

BASAL LAYER

In the epidermis, the short stacks of lipid lamellae that are extruded from the membrane-coating granules fuse at the edges to produce multiple broad lipid sheets which fill most of the extracellular spaces of the stratum corneum; in keratinized oral epithelium, about 50% of the intercellular space of the stratum corneum is occupied by desmosomes (Schroeder, 1981), and the interdesmosomal regions are frequently dilated. Although the extruded membrane-coating granule contents fuse to form multiple broad lipid sheets in the intercellular spaces of the stratum corneum of this tissue, the number of individual lamellae in oral tissue is less than that observed in epidermis.

The major lipid classes present in epidermal and oral stratum corneum are similar (Law et al., 1995), but the proportions of these lipids differ, and there is nearly an order of magnitude difference in barrier function as judged by permeability to water. Lipid composition will also influence the organization of the barrier lipids.

Although multiple, broad, lamellar sheets are present in both epidermal and oral stratum corneum, the highly ordered appearance of the multiple lipid sheets seen in epidermal stratum corneum is not observed in oral stratum corneum. In the oral tissue, the interdesmosomal portions of the intercellular space tend to be dilated with a few broad lamellae at the periphery of the dilation and less well-organized lamellae and non-lamellar material, possibly consisting of desmosomal breakdown products, filling the center of the dilation.

In *non-keratinized oral epithelia* (see Fig. 8.2), the accumulation of lipids is less evident than in keratinized epithelia. As

**Figure 8.2** Diagram to show the major structural changes during maturation and formation of the permeability barrier in non-keratinized epithelium. Membrane-coating granules containing short stacks of lipid lamellae and electron-lucent material migrate to the superficial cell membrane of cells in the intermediate layer of the epithelium. The membrane of the granule fuses with the cell plasma membrane and the lamellate contents are extruded into the intercellular space as shown in the electron micrograph in the top right panel. We are grateful to Dr. Philip Wertz for providing the panel insert.

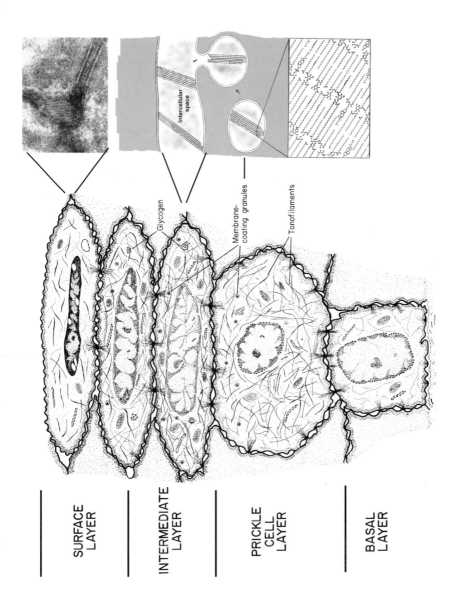

Glycogen

Membrane-
coating granules

Tonofilaments

Intercellular
space

SURFACE
LAYER

INTERMEDIATE
LAYER

PRICKLE
CELL
LAYER

BASAL
LAYER

cells reach the upper one-third to one-quarter of the epithelium, membrane-coating granules become evident at the
superficial aspect of the cells and appear to fuse with the
plasma membrane so as to extrude their contents into the
intercellular space. The membrane-coating granules found
in non-keratinizing epithelia are spherical in shape,
membrane-bounded, and measure about $0.2\,\mu m$ in diameter
(Squier, 1977). They have often been referred to as cored
granules because of their appearance in transmission electron micrographs of conventional, osmium tetroxide-fixed,
tissue. Such granules have been observed in a variety of
human non-keratinized epithelia, including oral mucosa,
uterine cervix (Grubb et al., 1968), and esophagus (Hopwood
et al., 1978). Only a small proportion of the granules in non-
keratinized epithelium contain lamellae, which may be the
source of short stacks of lamellar lipid scattered throughout
the intercellular spaces in the outer portion of the epithelium
(Wertz et al., 1993).

In contrast to the appearance of the intercellular spaces
of the surface layer of keratinized epithelia, those of the
superficial layer of non-keratinizing epithelia contain
electron-lucent material, which may represent non-lamellar
phase lipid, with only occasional short stacks of lipid lamellae. It is the absence of organized lipid lamellae in the intercellular spaces that accounts for the greater permeability of
this tissue. It seems likely that the lamellae seen in the intercellular spaces in the non-keratinizing epithelia are derived
from the lamellar material in the membrane-coating granules, and it is possible that these lamellae might have a lipid
composition distinctly different from the overall composition. If these structures are enriched in ceramides, cholesterol, and fatty acids and are well ordered, they could
account for much of the diffusional resistance of these tissues
to aqueous penetrants.

It is also noteworthy that epidermis and all of the oral epithelia synthesize appreciable quantities of glycosylceramides
(Squier et al., 1991) but differ in the extent of deglycosylation
in the formation of their barriers. In epidermis, where the
barrier is most effective, more than 98% of the sphingolipid in
the barrier was ceramide. In gingival and palatal stratum

corneum, 73% and 77%, respectively, of the sphingolipid had been converted to ceramides, whereas in the barriers from the buccal epithelium and the floor of the mouth, only about 5%–6% of the glycosylceramides had been converted.

## 8.1.1 Membrane-coating granules and the location of a permeability barrier in oral mucosa

Intercellular tracers such as horseradish peroxidase or lanthanum that can be visualized in the light or electron microscope have been used to demonstrate the location of the permeability barrier in oral mucosa (Squier, 1973; Squier and Rooney, 1976). In keratinized mucosa, the limit of penetration of the tracers was at the boundary of the granular and keratinized layers, as in epidermis. When the procedure was carried out using non-keratinized oral mucosa, the tracers failed to penetrate the outer one-third to one-quarter of the epithelium. This coincided with the level at which the membrane-coating granules of this tissue appear to fuse with the superficial cell membrane and extrude their contents into the intercellular space. Although these granules differ morphologically from those of keratinized epithelium, they appear to be homologous with the granules of keratinized epithelia in their location and behavior (Squier, 1977).

If the presence of membrane-coating granules in a stratified squamous epithelium is a prerequisite for the formation of a permeability barrier, then tissues from which they are absent might be expected to lack such a barrier. Epithelial cells from skin and keratinizing oral mucosa maintained in a submerged culture system show poor differentiation, and membrane-coating granules have rarely been described in ultrastructural studies. When such cultures are treated topically with horseradish peroxidase, it readily penetrates between the cells of the superficial layer, indicating that a permeability barrier is not present (Squier et al., 1978). The use of raised (interface) cultures has been found to facilitate epithelial differentiation, including the development of membrane-coating granules in epidermis (Madison et al.,

1988) and oral epithelium (Lillie et al., 1988). The permeability of such a system tends to be slightly higher than that of skin *in vivo* (Cumpstone et al., 1989), although equivalence has been reported (Cannon et al., 1994). Thus, in the junctional epithelium of the tooth, and in tissue culture systems, the presence or absence of membrane-coating granules can be related to the permeability properties of the tissue.

## 8.1.2 Other permeability barriers in oral mucosa

Although the superficial layers of the oral epithelium represent the primary barrier to the entry of substances from the exterior, it is evident that the basement membrane also plays a role in limiting the passage of materials across the junction between epithelium and connective tissue (Alfano et al., 1977). Thus, intravenously injected horseradish peroxidase can enter the intercellular spaces of the epidermis, but the passage of the larger molecules of the protein, thorotrast, is restricted (Wolff and Honigsmann, 1971). A similar mechanism appears to operate in the opposite direction. When labeled albumin is applied to the surface of the oral mucosa of animals sensitized to this protein, immune complexes that are formed in the epithelium are trapped above the basement membrane, suggesting that whereas immunoglobulins can traverse this region, the larger immunocomplexes do not (Tolo, 1974). The accumulation of materials in the basal region may represent the nonspecific binding of charged molecules to components of the basal lamina.

## 8.1.3 Aging and the permeability of oral mucosa

As discussed in Chapter 7, the oral mucosa shows few changes that can be unambiguously ascribed to aging. In some regions, there is a slight thinning of the epithelium with a concomitant flattening of the epithelial–connective tissue interface (Williams and Cruchley, 1994). The limited information available on the permeability of oral mucosa indicates that there is a trend toward decreased permeability to water with age which is statistically significant for floor of mouth mucosa from females (Squier et al., 1994). It is of interest to note that in skin, where the morphological changes with age are more marked than in oral mucosa, there have been a number of reports which demonstrate a significant decrease in permeability with age; the reasons for this have been discussed by Squier et al. (1994).

## 8.1.4 The permeability barrier and reactive changes in the oral mucosa

### Inflammation

The most common mucosal reaction to insult or disease is inflammation. The abundant vasculature ensures rapid infiltration of the tissue with inflammatory cells in response to mechanical or chemical insult. A mild degree of inflammation stimulates epithelial proliferation, leading to hyperplastic changes, whereas severe inflammation suppresses proliferation (Johnson, 1994) so that the epithelium may become thinner or even be lost (i.e., ulcerated).

A common site for mucosal inflammation is under dentures. Riber and Kaaber (1980) found inflammatory changes of the palatal mucosa after 12 months in one-third of a group of denture wearers. Permeability measurements on the inflamed tissue under the dentures revealed a threefold increase in permeability as compared to values for normal palate (Riber and Kaaber, 1978). This effect seemed to be associated with a shift in epithelial differentiation in the presence of chronic inflammation toward that of non-keratinization with a concomitant increase in permeability.

## 8.1.5 Permeability barrier function and extrinsic factors

A variety of extrinsic factors can bring about changes in the oral mucosa that have a potential for altering permeability. The most frequent of these is irritation from physical damage or from chemical irritants such as tobacco and tobacco smoke, alcohol, toothpastes, and mouth rinses. Assuming that inflammation is not severe (see previous section), oral epithelium responds to irritation by an increase in cell proliferation that results in a thickening of the tissue; keratinized regions tend to show a thickening of the keratinized layer (hyperkeratinization), and non-keratinized regions frequently develop a keratinized layer in these circumstances. The most dramatic hyperkeratotic changes in the oral mucosa are seen in the palate of smokers and at sites in the mouth such as the cheek, inner lip, and gums, where users of snuff or chewing tobacco place the product. These reactive changes presumably offer greater mechanical protection to the tissue but do not appear to improve its barrier properties. Indeed, hyperkeratotic hamster cheek pouch, induced by chemical or mechanical means, shows permeability values that are either no different from, or are greater than, normal tissue (Squier and Hall, 1985). Such findings are consistent with data from skin, where the thickened epidermis of the palmar and plantar regions has a higher permeability than thin skin (Kligman, 1964) and where the pathological thickening that is evident in conditions such as psoriasis and in various ichthyoses, results in an increased permeability to water (Grice, 1980). The reduced barrier function in conditions of epithelial thickening is probably a reflection of the increased cell proliferation and faster epithelial transit time characteristic of hyperplasia; this reduces the opportunity for membrane granule extrusion and adequate formation of the intercellular barrier material.

## 8.2 IMMUNOLOGIC BARRIER FUNCTION OF ORAL MUCOSA

Microorganisms in food, water, and air are a formidable challenge to the oral lining. At times, oral mucosal surfaces are exposed to high concentrations of environmental microorganisms and/or their products in respirable air, saprophytic microorganisms on foodstuffs, and microorganisms in water. Microorganisms residing in the oral cavity are also a burden; there are more than 500 diverse phylotypes of bacteria present in saliva (approximately $10^8$ microorganisms/ mL) and dental plaque (approximately $10^{11}$ microorganisms/ gram) (Aas et al., 2005). Oral tissues respond to the continual exposure to these microorganisms by creating immunologic barriers via innate and adaptive immune responses. This limits local infection, colonization, invasion, and inflammation by potential pathogens. The immunologic barrier defined by the innate immune response is prominent and consists of antimicrobial peptides, antimicrobial proteins, chemokines, cytokines, and neuropeptides, which are found in the oral tissues, saliva, and gingival crevicular fluid.

*Antimicrobial peptides* are small, potent molecules composed of anionic or cationic amino acid residues with broad spectrum antibiotic-like activities (Brogden, 2005). They also have many ancillary innate and adaptive immune functions (Yang et al., 2004). Antimicrobial peptides differ in size, amino acid residue composition, and mechanism of antimicrobial activity. These peptides are expressed in many tissues of the oral cavity. They have potent antimicrobial activity, neutralize lipopolysaccharide, promote wound healing, and have synergistic activity with conventional antibiotics. *Antimicrobial proteins* are larger and contain more than 100 amino acid residues, are often lytic enzymes, nutrient-binding proteins, or they contain sites that target specific microbial macromolecules (Ganz, 2003). Examples include lactoferrin and lysozyme; both are found in saliva and gingival crevicular fluid. *Cytokines* and *chemokines* have important roles in regulating and directing both innate and adaptive immune responses. *Neuropeptides* are peptides with neural or neuroendocrine signaling functions. Interestingly, some cytokines, chemokines, and neuropeptides also have direct antimicrobial activity contributing to the innate immune response barrier (Brogden et al., 2005).

## 8.2.1 Antimicrobial peptides and immune mediators in oral tissues

Oral tissues, including salivary glands, produce antimicrobial peptides, antimicrobial proteins, cytokines, and chemokines. The specific expression profiles for cells isolated from oral tissues are listed in Table 8.1. mRNA for human β-defensin 1 is strongly expressed in the broad spinous cell region and localized throughout the nucleated layers of the epithelium (Dale et al., 2001), and the peptide is present in the well-differentiated cells of the upper spinous and granular layers. mRNA for human β-defensin 2 is induced in the spinous and granular layers of the epithelium, and the peptide is present in the upper granular layers of epithelium with spotty presence in the spinous layers. Human β-defensin 3 is expressed in the basal layer in healthy tissue, occasionally extending into the spinous layers and upper layers (Lu et al., 2005). Human neutrophil peptide (HNP) α-defensins 1–3 and the cathelicidin LL-37 are both found in polymorphonuclear leukocytes in the connective tissue and junctional epithelium (Dale et al., 2001).

Myeloid dendritic cells produce a great variety of cytokines involved in T-helper (Th) cell responses for cell-mediated immunity (Th1 cytokines), humoral immunity (Th2 cytokines), autoimmunity and inflammation (Th17 cytokines), proinflammatory cytokines, anti-inflammatory cytokines, and chemokines. Human gingival epithelial cells, keratinocytes, and oral fibroblasts produce a lesser variety of proinflammatory cytokines and chemokines. Polymorphonuclear leukocytes can also produce cytokines, generally in response to inflammatory stimuli (Kasama et al., 2005).

## 8.2.2 Antimicrobial peptides and immune mediators in oral secretions

Many of the antimicrobial peptides, cytokines, and chemokines produced by oral tissues and salivary glands are present in saliva and gingival crevicular fluid (Table 8.2) and to a lesser extent in gingiva around implants and in dentinal fluid. Saliva is complex and contains over 1050 proteins (Hu et al., 2007) involved in oral lubrication, mastication, and digestion; innate immune defense of oral tissues; and demineralization and remineralization of teeth (Schenkels et al.,

**Table 8.1** Prominent mediators produced by individual cells in the oral cavity.

| | Epithelial cells[a] | Keratinocytes[b] | Fibroblasts[c] | Myeloid dendritic cells[d] | Polymorphonuclear leukocytes[e] |
|---|---|---|---|---|---|
| Antimicrobial peptides | | | | | |
| HNP (1,2,3) | | | | ✓ | ✓ |
| human β-defensin 1, 2, 3 | ✓ | ✓ | | | |
| LL-37 | ✓ | ✓ | | | ✓ |
| Th1 cytokines | | | | | |
| IFN-γ | | | | ✓ | |
| IL-2 | | ✓ | | ✓ | |
| IL-12(p70) | | | | ✓ | |
| Th2 cytokines | | | | | |
| IL-3 | | | | ✓ | |
| IL-4 | | | | ✓ | |
| IL-5 | | | | ✓ | |
| IL-10 | | | | ✓ | |
| IL-13 | | | | ✓ | |
| Th17 cytokines | | | | | |
| IL-17 | | ✓ | | ✓ | |
| IL-23 | | | | ✓ | |
| IFN-γ | | | | | |
| Proinflammatory cytokines | | | | | |
| Granulocyte-macrophage colony-stimulating factor (GM-CSF) | | | | | |

*(Continued)*

**Table 8.1** (Continued)

| | Epithelial cells[a] | Keratinocytes[b] | Fibroblasts[c] | Myeloid dendritic cells[d] | Polymorphonuclear leukocytes[e] |
|---|---|---|---|---|---|
| IL-1α | √ | √ | | √ | |
| IL-1β | | √ | | √ | √ |
| IL-12 | | √ | | √ | |
| IL-12(p40) | | | | √ | |
| IL-18 | √ | √ | √ | √ | √ |
| IL-6 | | √ | √ | √ | √ |
| TNF-α | | √ | | √ | |
| Anti-inflammatory cytokines | | | | | |
| IL-10 | | √ | √ | | |
| IL-13 | | | | | |
| TGF-β | | √ | | | |
| Chemokines | | | | | |
| CXCL3/GRO-ã | √ | √ | √ | √ | |
| CXCL8/IL-8 | | √ | √ | √ | √ |
| CXCL9/MIG | | √ | √ | √ | |
| CXCL10/IP-10 | | √ | √ | √ | |
| CXCL11/I-TAC | | √ | √ | √ | |
| CCL2/MCP-1 | | √ | | √ | √ |
| CCL3/MIP-1α | | | | √ | √ |
| CCL4/MIP-1β | | √ | | √ | |
| CCL5/RANTES | | | √ | √ | √ |

| | | |
|---|---|---|
| CCL11/eotaxin | | |
| Angiogenic factor | | |
| VEGF | √ | √ |
| GammaC family cytokines | | |
| IL-2 | √ | √ |
| IL-7 | √ | √ |
| IL-15 | √ | √ |

[a]Diamond et al. (2001), and Krisanaprakornkit et al. (1998).

[b]Bickel et al. (1996), Formanek et al. (1999), Joly et al. (2005), Mathews et al. (1999), Ohta et al. (2008), and Xu et al. (2009).

[c]Imatani et al. (2001), Ohta et al. (2008), Scheres et al. (2010), and Yamaji et al. (1995).

[d]Cutler and Teng (2007), and Pingel et al. (2008).

[e]Allstaedt et al. (1996), Gudmundsson et al. (1996), Kasama et al. (2005), and Rodriguez-Garcia et al. (2010).

**Table 8.2** Presence of antimicrobial innate defense molecules in the saliva and gingival crevicular fluid.

| Peptide/protein | Saliva[a] | Gingival crevicular fluid[b] |
|---|---|---|
| Neuropeptides | | |
| Adrenomedullin, substance P, neuropeptide Y, vasoactive intestinal peptide | 0.06–41.4 pg/mL | 0.061–1.8 µg/mL |
| Cationic antimicrobial peptides | | |
| HNP (1, 2, 3) | 0.1–39.2 µg/mL | 0.01–116.2 µg/mL |
| human β-defensin 1, 2, 3 | 0.0–7.3 µg/mL | Present |
| LL-37 | 1.6 µg/mL | 11 µg/mL |
| Histatins | 6–122 µg/mL | |
| Other peptides with antimicrobial activity | | |
| Statherin | 69.0 µg/mL | Present |
| β-2-microglobulin | | 9.4 µg/mL |
| CCL28 (mucosa-associated epithelial chemokine) | Present | |
| Azurocidin (CAP37) | Present | |
| Calcitonin gene-related peptide | Present | 0.013–0.7 µg/mL |
| Mucins (MG1,MG2) | 40 µg/mL | |
| Surfactant protein (A) | 0.9 µg/mL | |
| Acidic proline-rich peptides (PRP1-4, PC) | 51–81 µg/mL | Present |
| Fibronectin | Present | 106 µg/mL |
| Calgranulin (A, B) | 1.9 µg/mL | 240 µg/mL |
| Calprotectin | | 570 µg/mL |
| Psoriasin | Present | |
| Lactoferrin | 10–22 µg/mL | 600 µg/mL |
| Cystatins (A, B, C, D, S, SA, SN) | 0–116 µg/mL | 1.15 µg/mL |
| Secretory leukocyte protease inhibitor (SLPI) | 2.9 µg/mL | Present |
| Elafin | 0.02 µg/mL | |
| Lactoperoxidase | 1.9 µg/mL | Present |
| Myeloperoxidase | 3 µg/mL | 0.3–5.5 µg/mL |
| Lysozyme | 2–80 µg/mL | Present |

[a]Dale et al., (2006); Dawidson et al., (1997); Devine, (2003); Gardner et al., (2009); Ghosh et al., (2007); Gorr, (2009); Gusman et al., (2004); Pisano et al., (2005); Schenkels et al., (1995); and Tenovuo et al., (1987).

[b]Awawdeh et al., (2002); Diamond et al., (2001); Friedman et al., (1983); Gorr, (2009); Kaner et al., (2006); Kido et al., (1999); Linden et al., (1997); Lundy et al., (2000, 2005, 2006); Pisano et al., (2005); and Suomalainen et al., (1996).

1995). Acidic proline-rich proteins have a high affinity for hydroxyapatite, inhibit crystal growth of calcium phosphate salts from solutions supersaturated with respect to hydroxyapatite, and bind calcium ions. Statherins, histatins, and cystatins inhibit calcium phosphate precipitation. Acidic proline-rich proteins, lysozyme, lactoferrin, HNP α-defensins, human β-defensins, cathelicidins, and histatins have antimicrobial activities. The defensins, cathelicidins, and histatins participate in various aspects of innate immunity (Yang et al., 2004), and the defensins, cathelicidins, and lactoferrin have immunomodulatory and antitumor activities. Insulin-like growth factor I and TGF-α in saliva stimulate the regeneration of tissue, induce the expression of antimicrobial peptides, and have additional immunologic functions (Kumar et al., 1995).

Saliva contains Th1 cytokines (IL-2, IL-12, and interferon-gamma [IFNγ]), Th2 cytokines (IL-4 and IL-10), proinflammatory cytokines (IL-1, IL-6, and TNF-α), and chemokines (CXCL8/IL-8, CCL2/MCP-1, CCL3/MIP-1 α, and CCL5/RANTES).

Saliva contains mucins with antimicrobial activity. Human salivary mucin glycoprotein MG1 binds to *Haemophilus parainfluenzae* (Veerman et al., 1995), human salivary mucin glycoprotein MG2 acts against oral microbial species (Antonyraj et al., 1998), and extra parotid glycoprotein (EP-GP) is a 20-kDa glycoprotein that binds selectively to strains of *Streptococcus salivarius* (Schenkels et al., 1997).

Gingival crevicular fluid is a serum transudate in the gingival sulcus bathing normal gingival tissues. It is rich in growth factors, antimicrobial peptides, serum proteins, and neuropeptides (Table 8.2). The volume of gingival crevicular fluid can vary, and sites characterized as being moderately or severely inflamed have a greater volume of gingival crevicular fluid than less inflamed sites (Lamster and Ahlo, 2007; Thunell et al., 2010). Concentrations of chemokines, proinflammatory cytokines, antimicrobial proteins, antimicrobial peptides, host-derived enzymes and their inhibitors, inflammatory mediators, host-response modifiers, and by-products of tissue breakdown are all elevated in moderately or severely inflamed sites.

Fluid in the gingival cuff around dental implants is similar in composition to gingival crevicular fluid. Human β-defensin 1 and human β-defensin 2 are both produced (Kuula et al., 2008). Dentinal fluid is a transudate extracellular fluid within the dentin that originates from odontoblastic processes. mRNA for human β-defensin 1 and human β-defensin 2, possibly produced by odontoblasts (Dommisch et al., 2005) and low levels of IL-6 and IL-8 are present.

## 8.2.3 Specific antimicrobial peptides in oral tissues and secretions

HNP α-defensins, human β-defensins, cathelicidins, lactoferrin, lysozyme, and histatins are among the dominant antimicrobial peptides expressed in oral tissues, saliva, and gingival crevicular fluid (Gorr, 2009). They have antimicrobial activity against gram-negative bacteria, gram-positive bacteria, fungi, and some viruses. There is variability in antimicrobial activity, and periodontopathogens can be more resistant to antimicrobial peptides than other oral bacteria (Joly et al., 2004).

HNP α-defensins are produced by salivary glands and by polymorphonuclear leukocytes in the sulcular and junctional epithelium (Dale et al., 2001; Lundy et al., 2004). They are present in saliva and gingival crevicular fluid (Table 8.2). HNP α-defensins contain 29–33 amino acid residues and have broad antimicrobial activities (Rehaume and Hancock, 2008). They are very similar in size and amino acid composition: HNP-1 has an additional N-terminal alanine residue; HNP-3 has an additional N-terminal aspartic acid residue; HNP-4 is slightly larger with more variability in its amino acid composition; and HNP-4 is rich in arginine (15.2 mol %) and is significantly more hydrophobic.

Human β-defensins are produced in the tongue (e.g., cells in the cornified tips of the filiform, but not fungiform, papillae), salivary glands, tonsils (e.g., surface epithelium and crypt epithelium), and nose (e.g., epithelial cell cytoplasm of the maxillary sinus mucosa). Human β-defensins are produced in the oral epithelium and sulcular epithelium (Dale et al., 2001); they are also present in saliva and gingival crevicular fluid (Table 8.2).

Human β-defensins vary in size, amino acid composition, and cationic charge (Selsted and Ouellette, 2005). Human β-defensin 1 contains 36 amino acid residues with a +3 charge, and human β-defensin 2 contains 42 amino acid residues with a +7 charge. Human β-defensin 3 contains 45 amino acid residues, has a β-sheet structure in solution, forms dimers, and has a +11 charge.

Cathelicidins are a family of peptides defined by a common N-terminal preproregion of about 100 residues that is homologous to the cysteine protease inhibitor cathelin (Zanetti, 2004). In humans, the active cathelicidin is LL-37. The mature peptide contains 37 amino acid residues. LL-37 is produced in the airways (e.g., squamous epithelia), mouth, tongue, tonsils (e.g., surface epithelium and crypt epithelium), and salivary glands (e.g., glandular epithelium) and is produced by polymorphonuclear leukocytes in the connective tissue and sulcular and junctional epithelium (Dale et al., 2001).

Lactoferrin is a member of the transferrin family of iron-binding proteins, is approximately 80 kDa in size, and has two iron-binding sites per molecule. It is present in saliva, nasal secretions, gingival crevicular fluid, and polymorphonuclear leukocytes secondary granules. It plays a role in iron uptake, is antimicrobial, is involved in phagocytic killing and in immune responses, serves as a growth factor, and prevents biofilm development (Lonnerdal and Iyer, 1995; Singh et al., 2002).

Lysozyme is a 14-KDa cationic enzyme secreted by macrophages and is found in the primary azurophil and secondary specific granules of polymorphonuclear leukocytes (Ganz et al., 1986). It is in saliva, nasal secretions, and gingival crevicular fluid (Table 8.2). It is bactericidal and cleaves the glycosidic bond between the two major repeating units, N-acetylmuramic acid and N-acetylglucosamine of the bacterial cell wall peptidoglycan (Chipman and Sharon, 1969).

Histatins are produced by the human parotid, submandibular, and sublingual salivary glands. There are 12 related peptides, all cationic and rich in histidine, lysine, and arginine amino acid residues. In fact, with the exception of an occasional amino acid substitution, all 12 family members appear as smaller congeners of histatin 1, histatin 3, or histatin 5 (Tsai and Bobek, 1998). They have broad spectrum antimicrobial activity against bacteria and fungi.

Some neuropeptides and peptide hormones are present in saliva and gingival crevicular fluids, suggesting that the nervous system may be directly involved in innate immune barrier defense of the oral cavity (Brogden et al., 2005). Substance P, neuropeptide Y, and adrenomedullin are found in saliva and gingival crevicular fluid, and have antimicrobial activity against multiple microbial species, including many oral microorganisms. Neuropeptides, like substance P, are involved in other aspects of innate defense by binding to NK1 receptors on junctional epithelial cells, endothelial cells, polymorphonuclear leukocytes, and monocytes. This induces infiltration of polymorphonuclear leukocytes from blood vessels into the junctional epithelium, cytokine production by monocytes, and increases permeability of blood vessels beneath the junctional epithelium.

Human salivary mucin glycoproteins MG1, human salivary mucin glycoprotein MG2, and extra parotid glycoprotein (EP-GP) bind and are antimicrobial against oral microbial species. However, the role of mucin and glycoprotein binding to bacterial cells in protection against infection is not yet known.

## 8.2.4 Induction and regulation of antimicrobial peptides

Microorganisms and microbial products induce the production of defensins through receptors on the cell surface. These receptors, called Toll-like receptors (TLR), recognize distinct repertoires of conserved microbial molecules (Froy, 2005). Binding and activation of the TLRs initiate an array of intracellular signaling pathways, including specific kinase pathways like the mitogen-activated protein kinase (MAPK) pathway or nuclear factor kappa-light-chain-enhancer of activated B cells (NF-κB) pathway. Both culminate in a proinflammatory response that involves the secretion of cytokines, chemokines, and defensins. The MAPK pathway is mediated by three protein kinases that phosphorylate and activate one another. The extracellular signal-regulated kinases (ERKs) control cell division, the c-Jun amino-terminal kinases (JNKs) regulate transcription, and the p38 kinases control cellular responses to cytokines and stress. The outcome of triggering is often dependent upon the specific microorganism or microbial product. For example, human gingival epithelial cells exposed to *Escherichia coli* and *Fusobacterium nucleatum* express human β-defensin 2, human β-defensin 3, and IL-8 whereas human gingival epithelial cells exposed to *Porphyromonas gingivalis* express human β-defensin 1 and human β-defensin 3 (Krisanaprakornkit et al., 2000). TLR2 and TLR4 induce expression of human β-defensin 2 by lipopolysaccharide or peptidoglycan, which occurs via the JNK pathway; TLR5 induces expression of human β-defensin 2 by *Salmonella enteritidis* flagellin, which occurs via the p38 and ERK pathways, and expression of human β-defensin 2 by *F. nucleatum*, which occurs via the p38 and JNK pathways. Expression of human β-defensin 3 occurs via the p38 and epidermal growth factor receptor (EGFR)/ERK pathways (Sorensen et al., 2005).

Cytokines induce the production of defensins (Joly et al., 2005; Kolls et al., 2008). Keratinocytes exposed to IFN-γ produce human β-defensin 1; keratinocytes exposed to IFN-γ and TNF-α or IL-1β and TNF-α produce human β-defensin 2; and keratinocytes exposed to IFN-γ or IFN-γ and TNF-α produce human β-defensin 3.

Conversely, defensins also induce the production of cytokines and chemokines (Boniotto et al., 2006; Niyonsaba et al., 2007). In keratinocytes and peripheral blood mononuclear cells, human β-defensins 1, 2, 3, and 4 induce the cytokines IL-1β, IL-6, IL-10, IL-18, and the chemokines CCL2/MCP-1, CCL4/MIP-1β, CCL5/RANTES, CCL8/MCP-2, CCL20/MIP-3α, CXCL3/GRO, CXCL8/IL-8, and CXCL10/IP-10.

Defensins induce the production of cytokines and chemokines via a variety of signaling pathways (Niyonsaba et al., 2007; Stroinigg and Srivastava, 2005; Yang et al., 1999).

Human β-defensin 2 activates dendritic cells via CCR6 or colon and breast cells via TLR7 resulting in activation of NF-κB, STAT1, STAT3, p38, and ERK 1/2 MAPK pathways. Human β-defensin 3 activates dendritic cells via TLR1 and 2 resulting in signaling that requires Myeloid Differentiation Factor 88 (MyD88) and results in IL-1 receptor-associated kinase-1 phosphorylation (Funderburg et al., 2007). Finally, defensins can even induce the production of other antimicrobial peptides like LL-37 (Stroinigg and Srivastava, 2005).

## 8.2.5 Innate and adaptive immune properties of antimicrobial peptides

Defensins have potent, concentration-dependent, innate, and adaptive immune functions (Yang et al., 2004). At low concentrations of 0.1–500 ng/mL, HNP α-defensins and human β-defensins attract and activate monocytes, macrophages, T lymphocytes, mast cells, and immature dendritic cells. At intermediate concentrations of 0.1–10 μg/mL, defensins have anti-inflammatory properties, adjuvant-like properties for co-administered antigens, and enhance the proliferation of epithelial cells. At higher concentrations of 2–40 μg/mL, defensins induce the production of cytokines and chemokines. At or above 50 μg/mL, HNP α-defensins and human β-defensins are cytotoxic.

LL-37 modulates innate and adaptive immune responses. It chemoattracts T lymphocytes, monocytes, mast cells, and polymorphonuclear leukocytes by its interaction with the formyl-methionine-leucine-phenylalanine (fMLP) receptor, a G-protein-coupled receptor (Zanetti, 2004). It inhibits macrophage activation by bacterial products: lipopolysaccharide, lipoteichoic acid, and lipoarabinomannan (Scott et al., 2002). LL-37 directly upregulates genes encoding chemokines and chemokine receptors, particularly for the expression of chemokines CCL2/MCP-1 and CXCL8/IL-8 and chemokine receptors CXCR-4, CCR2, and IL-8RB (Scott et al., 2002). LL-37 enhances an antitumor immune response to $CSFR_{J6-1}$ (macrophage colony-stimulating factor receptor cloned from the J6-1 leukemic cell line) (An et al., 2005).

Histatins have a variety of putative biological functions (Tsai and Bobek, 1998). In addition to direct antimicrobial activity against oral bacteria and fungi, histatins can bind to oral microorganisms, neutralize toxins (e.g., *Aggregatibacter actinomycetemcomitans* RTX toxin), inactivate protease and collagenase activities, inhibit hemagglutinating activity of *P. gingivalis* and *Tannerella forsythensis*; inhibit co-aggregation of oral bacteria; inhibit lipopolysaccharide-mediated activities; and induce histamine release from mast cells.

In conclusion, the oral tissues respond to the continual exposure of microorganisms by creating an immunologic barrier of antimicrobial peptides, antimicrobial proteins, chemokines, cytokines, and neuropeptides. These mediators limit infection and inflammation directly and via activation of other innate and adaptive immune responses.

# REFERENCES

Aas, J.A., Paster, B.J., Stokes, L.N., Olsen, I., and Dewhirst, F.E. (2005) Defining the normal bacterial flora of the oral cavity. J Clin Microbiol 43:5721–5732.

Alfano, M.C., Chasen, A.E., and Masi, C.W. (1977) Autoradiographic study of the penetration of radiolabelled dextrans and inulin through non-keratinized oral mucosa in vitro. J Periodont Res 12:368–377.

Altstaedt, J., Kirchner, H., and Rink, L. (1996) Cytokine production of neutrophils is limited to interleukin-8. Immunology 89:563–568.

An, L.L., Yang, Y.H., Ma, X.T., Lin, Y.M., Li, G., Song, Y.H., and Wu, K.F. (2005) LL-37 enhances adaptive antitumor immune response in a murine model when genetically fused with M-CSFR (J6-1) DNA vaccine. Leuk Res 29:535–543.

Antonyraj, K.J., Karunakaran, T., and Raj, P.A. (1998) Bactericidal activity and poly-L-proline II conformation of the tandem repeat sequence of human salivary mucin glycoprotein (MG2). Arch Biochem Biophys 356:197–206.

Awawdeh, L.A., Lundy, F.T., Linden, G.J., Shaw, C., Kennedy, J.G., and Lamey, P.J. (2002) Quantitative analysis of substance P, neurokinin A and calcitonin gene-related peptide in gingival crevicular fluid associated with painful human teeth. Eur J Oral Sci 110:185–191.

Bickel, M., Nothen, S.M., Freiburghaus, K., and Shire, D. (1996) Chemokine expression in human oral keratinocyte cell lines and keratinized mucosa. J Dent Res 75:1827–1834.

Boniotto, M., Jordan, W.J., Eskdale, J., Tossi, A., Antcheva, N., Crovella, S., Connell, N.D., and Gallagher, G. (2006) Human beta-defensin 2 induces a vigorous cytokine response in peripheral blood mononuclear cells. Antimicrob Agents Chemother 50:1433–1441.

Brogden, K.A. (2005) Antimicrobial peptides: pore formers or metabolic inhibitors in bacteria? Nat Rev Microbiol 3:238–250.

Brogden, K.A., Guthmiller, J.M., Salzet, M., and Zasloff, M. (2005) The nervous system and innate immunity: the neuro-peptide connection. Nat Immunol 6:558–564.

Cannon, C.L., Neal, P.J., Kubilus, J., Klausner, M., Swartzendruber, D.C., Squier, C.A., Kremer, M.J., and Wertz, P.W. (1994) Lipid and ultrastructural characterization of a new epidermal model shows good correspondence to normal human epidermis. J Invest Dermatol 102:600.

Chipman, D.M., and Sharon, N. (1969) Mechanism of lysozyme action. Science 165:454–465.

Cumpstone, N.B., Kennedy, A.H., Hannon, C.S., and Potts, R.O. (1989) The water permeability of primary mouse keratino-cyte cultures grown at the air-liquid interface. J Invest Dermatol 92:598.

Cutler, C.W., and Teng, Y.T. (2007) Oral mucosal dendritic cells and periodontitis: many sides of the same coin with new twists. Periodontology 2000(45):35–50.

Dale, B.A., Kimball, J.R., Krisanaprakornkit, S., Roberts, F., Robinovitch, M., O'Neal, R., Valore, E.V., Ganz, T., Anderson, G.M., and Weinberg, A. (2001) Localized antimicrobial peptide expression in human gingiva. J Periodontal Res 36:285–294.

Dale, B.A., Tao, R., Kimball, J.R., and Jurevic, R.J. (2006) Oral antimicrobial peptides and biological control of caries. BMC Oral Health 6:S13.

Dawidson, I., Blom, M., Lundeberg, T., Theodorsson, E., and Angmar-Mansson, B. (1997) Neuropeptides in the saliva of healthy subjects. Life Sci 60:269–278.

Devine, D.A. (2003) Antimicrobial peptides in defence of the oral and respiratory tracts. Mol Immunol 40:431–443.

Diamond, D.L., Kimball, J.R., Krisanaprakornkit, S., Ganz, T., and Dale, B.A. (2001) Detection of β-defensins secreted by human oral epithelial cells. J Immunol Methods 256:65–76.

Dommisch, H., Winter, J., Acil, Y., Dunsche, A., Tiemann, M., and Jepsen, S. (2005) Human beta-defensin (hBD-1, -2) expression in dental pulp. Oral Microbiol Immunol 20:163–166.

Formanek, M., Knerer, B., and Kornfehl, J. (1999) Cytokine expression of human oral keratinocytes. ORL J Otorhinolaryngol Relat Spec 61:103–107.

Friedman, S.A., Mandel, I.D., and Herrera, M.S. (1983) Lysozyme and lactoferrin quantitation in the crevicular fluid. J Periodontol 54:347–350.

Froy, O. (2005) Regulation of mammalian defensin expression by Toll-like receptor-dependent and independent signalling pathways. Cell Microbiol 7:1387–1397.

Funderburg, N., Lederman, M.M., Feng, Z., Drage, M.G., Jadlowsky, J., Harding, C.V., Weinberg, A., and Sieg, S.F. (2007) Human β-defensin-3 activates professional antigen-presenting cells via Toll-like receptors 1 and 2. Proc Natl Acad Sci U S A 104:18631–18635.

Ganz, T. (2003) The role of antimicrobial peptides in innate immunity. Integr Comp Biol 43:300–304.

Ganz, T., Selsted, M.E., and Lehrer, R.I. (1986) Antimicrobial activity of phagocyte granule proteins. Semin Respir Infect 1:107–117.

Gardner, M.S., Rowland, M.D., Siu, A.Y., Bundy, J.L., Wagener, D.K., and Stephenson, J.L. (2009) Comprehensive defensin assay for saliva. Anal Chem 81:557–566.

Ghosh, S.K., Gerken, T.A., Schneider, K.M., Feng, Z., McCormick, T.S., and Weinberg, A. (2007) Quantification of human beta-defensin-2 and -3 in body fluids: application for studies of innate immunity. Clin Chem 53:757–765.

Gorr, S.U. (2009) Antimicrobial peptides of the oral cavity. Periodontology 2000(51):152–180.

Grice, R.A. (1980) Transepidermal water loss in pathological skin. In: The Physiology and Pathophysiology of the Skin (A. Jarrett, ed.) p. 2147. Academic Press, London.

Grubb, C., Hackemann, M., and Hill, K.R. (1968) Small granules and plasma membrane thickening in human cervical squamous epithelium. J Ultrastruct Res 22:258–268.

Gudmundsson, G.H., Agerberth, B., Odeberg, J., Bergman, T., Olsson, B., and Salcedo, R. (1996) The human gene FALL39 and processing of the cathelin precursor to the antibacterial peptide LL-37 in granulocytes. Eur J Biochem 238:325–332.

Gusman, H., Leone, C., Helmerhorst, E.J., Nunn, M., Flora, B., Troxler, R.F., and Oppenheim, F.G. (2004) Human salivary gland-specific daily variations in histatin concentrations determined by a novel quantitation technique. Arch Oral Biol 49:11–22.

Hopwood, D., Logan, K.R., and Bouchier, I.A.D. (1978) The electron microscopy of normal human oesophageal epithelium. Virchows Arch B Cell Pathol 26:345–358.

Hu, S., Loo, J.A., and Wong, D.T. (2007) Human saliva proteome analysis. Ann N Y Acad Sci 1098:323–329.

Imatani, T., Kato, T., and Okuda, K. (2001) Production of inflammatory cytokines by human gingival fibroblasts stimulated by cell-surface preparations of *Porphyromonas gingivalis*. Oral Microbiol Immunol 16:65–72.

Johnson, G.K. (1994) Effects of aging on the microvasculature and microcirculation in skin and oral mucosa. In: The Effect of Aging in Oral Mucosa and Skin (C.A. Squier and M.W. Hill, eds.) pp. 99–106. CRC Press, Boca Raton, FL.

Joly, S., Maze, C., McCray, P.B., Jr., and Guthmiller, J.M. (2004) Human beta-defensins 2 and 3 demonstrate strain-selective activity against oral microorganisms. J Clin Microbiol 42:1024–1029.

Joly, S., Organ, C.C., Johnson, G.K., McCray, P.B., Jr., and Guthmiller, J.M. (2005) Correlation between beta-defensin expression and induction profiles in gingival keratinocytes. Mol Immunol 42:1073–1084.

Kaner, D., Bernimoulin, J.P., Kleber, B.M., Heizmann, W.R., and Friedmann, A. (2006) Gingival crevicular fluid levels of calprotectin and myeloperoxidase during therapy for generalized aggressive periodontitis. J Periodontal Res 41:132–139.

Kasama, T., Miwa, Y., Isozaki, T., Odai, T., Adachi, M., and Kunkel, S.L. (2005) Neutrophil-derived cytokines: potential therapeutic targets in inflammation. Curr Drug Targets Inflamm Allergy 4:273–279.

Kido, J., Nakamura, T., Kido, R., Ohishi, K., Yamauchi, N., Kataoka, M., and Nagata, T. (1999) Calprotectin in gingival crevicular fluid correlates with clinical and biochemical markers of periodontal disease. J Clin Periodontol 26:653–657.

Kligman, M. (1964) The biology of the stratum corneum. In: The Epidermis (W. Montagna and W.C. Lobity, eds.) pp. 387–433. Academic Press, New York.

Kolls, J.K., McCray, P.B., Jr., and Chan, Y.R. (2008) Cytokine-mediated regulation of antimicrobial proteins. Nat Rev Immunol 8:829–835.

Krisanaprakornkit, S., Weinberg, A., Perez, C.N., and Dale, B.A. (1998) Expression of the peptide antibiotic human b-defensin 1 in cultured gingival epithelial cells and gingival tissue. Infect Immun 66:4222–4228.

Krisanaprakornkit, S., Kimball, J.R., Weinberg, A., Darveau, R.P., Bainbridge, B.W., and Dale, B.A. (2000) Inducible expression of human beta-defensin 2 by *Fusobacterium nucleatum* in oral epithelial cells: multiple signaling pathways and role of commensal bacteria in innate immunity and the epithelial barrier. Infect Immun 68:2907–2915.

Kumar, V., Bustin, S.A., and McKay, I.A. (1995) Transforming growth factor alpha. Cell Biol Int 19:373–388.

Kuula, H., Salo, T., Pirila, E., Hagstrom, J., Luomanen, M., Gutierrez-Fernandez, A., Romanos, G.E., and Sorsa, T. (2008) Human beta-defensin-1 and -2 and matrix metalloproteinase-25 and -26 expression in chronic and aggressive periodontitis and in peri-implantitis. Arch Oral Biol 53:175–186.

Lamster, I.B., and Ahlo, J.K. (2007) Analysis of gingival crevicular fluid as applied to the diagnosis of oral and systemic diseases. Ann N Y Acad Sci 1098:216–229.

Landmann, L. (1988) The epidermal permeability barrier. Anat Embryol 178:1–13.

Law, S., Wertz, P.W., Swartzendruber, D.C., and Squier, C.A. (1995) Regional variation in content, composition and organization of porcine epithelial barrier lipids revealed by thin-layer chromatography and transmission electron microscopy. Arch Oral Biol 40:1085–1091.

Lillie, J.H., MacCullum, D.K., and Jepsen, A. (1988) Growth of stratified squamous epithelium on reconstituted extracellular matrices: long-term culture. J Invest Dermatol 90:100–109.

Linden, G.J., McKinnell, J., Shaw, C., and Lundy, F.T. (1997) Substance P and neurokinin A in gingival crevicular fluid in periodontal health and disease. J Clin Periodontol 24:799–803.

Lonnerdal, B., and Iyer, S. (1995) Lactoferrin: molecular structure and biological function. Annu Rev Nutr 15:93–110.

Lu, Q., Samaranayake, L.P., Darveau, R.P., and Jin, L. (2005) Expression of human beta-defensin-3 in gingival epithelia. J Periodontal Res 40:474–481.

Lundy, F.T., Mullally, B.H., Burden, D.J., Lamey, P.J., Shaw, C., and Linden, G.J. (2000) Changes in substance P and neurokinin A in gingival crevicular fluid in response to periodontal treatment. J Clin Periodontol 27:526–530.

Lundy, F.T., Orr, D.F., Gallagher, J.R., Maxwell, P., Shaw, C., Napier, S.S., Gerald Cowan, C., Lamey, P.J., and Marley, J.J. (2004) Identification and overexpression of human neutrophil alpha-defensins (human neutrophil peptides 1, 2 and 3) in squamous cell carcinomas of the human tongue. Oral Oncol 40:139–144.

Lundy, F.T., Orr, D.F., Shaw, C., Lamey, P.J., and Linden, G.J. (2005) Detection of individual human neutrophil alpha-defensins (human neutrophil peptides 1, 2 and 3) in unfractionated gingival crevicular fluid—a MALDI-MS approach. Mol Immunol 42:575–579.

Lundy, F.T., O'Hare, M., McKibben, B.M., Fulton, C.R., Briggs, J.E., and Linden, G.J. (2006) Radioimmunoassay quantification of adrenomedullin in human gingival crevicular fluid. Arch Oral Biol 51:334–338.

Madison, K.C., Swartzendruber, D.C., Wertz, P.W., and Downing, D.T. (1988) Lamellar granule extrusion and stratum corneum intercellular lamellae in murine keratinocytes. J Invest Dermatol 90:110–116.

Martinez, I.R., and Peters, A. (1971) Membrane-coating granules and membrane modifications in keratinizing epithelia. Am J Anat 130:93–119.

Mathews, M., Jia, H.P., Guthmiller, J.M., Losh, G., Graham, S., Johnson, G.K., Tack, B.F., and McCray, P.B., Jr. (1999) Production of b-defensin antimicrobial peptides by the oral mucosa and salivary glands. Infect Immun 67:2740–2745.

Niyonsaba, F., Ushio, H., Nakano, N., Ng, W., Sayama, K., Hashimoto, K., Nagaoka, I., Okumura, K., and Ogawa, H. (2007) Antimicrobial peptides human beta-defensins stimulate epidermal keratinocyte migration, proliferation and production of proinflammatory cytokines and chemokines. J Invest Dermatol 127:594–604.

Ohta, K., Shigeishi, H., Taki, M., Nishi, H., Higashikawa, K., Takechi, M., and Kamata, N. (2008) Regulation of CXCL9/10/11 in oral keratinocytes and fibroblasts. J Dent Res 87:1160–1165.

Pingel, L.C., Kohlgraf, K.G., Hansen, C.J., Eastman, C.G., Dietrich, D.E., Burnell, K.K., Srikantha, R.N., Xiao, X., Belanger, M., Progulske-Fox, A., Cavanaugh, J.E., Guthmiller, J.M., Johnson, G.K., Joly, S., Kurago, Z.B., Dawson, D.V., and Brogden, K.A. (2008) Human beta-defensin 3 binds to hemagglutinin B (rHagB), a non-fimbrial adhesin from *Porphyromonas gingivalis*, and attenuates a proinflammatory cytokine response. Immunol Cell Biol 86:643–649.

Pisano, E., Cabras, T., Montaldo, C., Piras, V., Inzitari, R., Olmi, C., Castagnola, M., and Messana, I. (2005) Peptides of human gingival crevicular fluid determined by HPLC-ESI-MS. Eur J Oral Sci 113:462–468.

Rehaume, L.M., and Hancock, R.E. (2008) Neutrophil-derived defensins as modulators of innate immune function. Crit Rev Immunol 28:185–200.

Riber, E., and Kaaber, S. (1978) Barrier properties of inflamed denture-loaded palatal mucosa to water. Scand J Dent Res 86:386–391.

Riber, E., and Kaaber, S. (1980) A 12-month study on changes in the barrier properties of denture-loaded palatal mucosa in immediate denture wearers. Scand J Dent Res 88:50–256.

Rodriguez-Garcia, M., Climent, N., Oliva, H., Casanova, V., Franco, R., Leon, A., Gatell, J.M., Garcia, F., and Gallart, T. (2010) Increased alpha-defensins 1-3 production by dendritic cells in HIV-infected individuals is associated with slower disease progression. PLoS ONE 5:e9436.

Schenkels, L.C., Veerman, E.C., and Nieuw Amerongen, A.V. (1995) Biochemical composition of human saliva in relation to other mucosal fluids. Crit Rev Oral Biol Med 6:161–175.

Schenkels, L.C., Walgreen-Weterings, E., Oomen, L.C., Bolscher, J.G., Veerman, E.C., and Nieuw Amerongen, A.V. (1997) In vivo binding of the salivary glycoprotein EP-GP (identical to GCDFP-15) to oral and non-oral bacteria detection and identification of EP-GP binding species. Biol Chem 378:83–88.

Scheres, N., Laine, M.L., de Vries, T.J., Everts, V., and van Winkelhoff, A.J. (2010) Gingival and periodontal ligament fibroblasts differ in their inflammatory response to viable *Porphyromonas gingivalis*. J Periodontal Res 45:262–270.

Schroeder, H.E. (1981) Differentiation of Human Oral Stratified Epithelium. Karger, Basel, pp. 35–156.

Scott, M.G., Davidson, D.J., Gold, M.R., Bowdish, D., and Hancock, R.E. (2002) The human antimicrobial peptide LL-37 is a multifunctional modulator of innate immune responses. J Immunol 169:3883–3891.

Selsted, M.E., and Ouellette, A.J. (2005) Mammalian defensins in the antimicrobial immune response. Nat Immunol 6:551–557.

Singh, P.K., Parsek, M.R., Greenberg, E.P., and Welsh, M.J. (2002) A component of innate immunity prevents bacterial biofilm development. Nature 417:552–555.

Sorensen, O.E., Thapa, D.R., Rosenthal, A., Liu, L., Roberts, A.A., and Ganz, T. (2005) Differential regulation of beta-defensin expression in human skin by microbial stimuli. J Immunol 174:4870–4879.

Squier, C.A. (1973) The permeability of keratinized and nonkeratinized oral epithelium to horseradish peroxidase. J Ultrastruct Res 43:160–177.

Squier, C.A. (1977) Membrane coating granules in nonkeratinized oral epithelium. J Ultrastruc Res 60:212–220.

Squier, C.A., and Hall, B.K. (1985) The permeability of hyperplastic oral epithelium. J Oral Pathol 14:357–362.

Squier, C.A., and Rooney, L. (1976) The permeability of keratinized and nonkeratinized oral epithelium to lanthanum in vivo. J Ultrastruct Res 54:286–295.

Squier, C.A., Fejerskov, O., and Jepsen, A. (1978) The permeability of a keratinizing squamous epithelium in culture. J Anat 126:103–109.

Squier, C.A., Cox, P., and Wertz, P.W. (1991) Lipid content and water permeability of skin and oral mucosa. J Invest Dermatol 96:123–126.

Squier, C.A., Wertz, P.W., Williams, D.M., and Cruchley, A.T. (1994) Permeability of oral mucosa and skin with age. In: The Effect of Aging in Oral Mucosa and Skin (C.A. Squier and M.W. Hill, eds.) pp. 91–98. CRC, Boca Raton, FL.

Stroinigg, N., and Srivastava, M.D. (2005) Modulation of toll-like receptor 7 and LL-37 expression in colon and breast epithelial cells by human beta-defensin-2. Allergy Asthma Proc 26:299–309.

Suomalainen, K., Saxen, L., Vilja, P., and Tenovuo, J. (1996) Peroxidases, lactoferrin and lysozyme in peripheral blood neutrophils, gingival crevicular fluid and whole saliva of patients with localized juvenile periodontitis. Oral Dis 2:129–134.

Tenovuo, J., Grahn, E., Lehtonen, O.P., Hyyppa, T., Karhuvaara, L., and Vilja, P. (1987) Antimicrobial factors in saliva: ontogeny and relation to oral health. J Dent Res 66:475–479.

Thunell, D.H., Tymkiw, K.D., Johnson, G.K., Joly, S., Burnell, K.K., Cavanaugh, J.E., Brogden, K.A., and Guthmiller, J.M. (2010) A multiplex immunoassay demonstrates reductions in gingival crevicular fluid cytokines following initial periodontal therapy. J Periodontal Res 45:148–152. JRE-05-08-0649.R1.

Tolo, K.J. (1974) Penetration of human albumin through oral mucosa of guinea pigs immunized to this protein. Arch Oral Biol 19:259–263.

Tsai, H., and Bobek, L.A. (1998) Human salivary histatins: promising anti-fungal therapeutic agents. Crit Rev Oral Biol Med 9:480–497.

Veerman, E.C., Ligtenberg, A.J., Schenkels, L.C., Walgreen-Weterings, E., and Nieuw Amerongen, A.V. (1995) Binding of human high-molecular-weight salivary mucins (MG1) to *Haemophilus parainfluenzae*. J Dent Res 74:351–357.

Wertz, P.W., Swartzendruber, D.C., and Squier, C.A. (1993) Regional variation in the structure and permeability of oral mucosa and skin. Adv Drug Deliv Rev 12:1–12.

Williams, D.M., and Cruchley, A.R. (1994) Structural aspects of aging in the oral mucosa. In: The Effect of Aging in Oral Mucosa and Skin (C.A. Squier and M.W. Hill, eds.) pp. 65–74. CRC Press, Boca Raton, FL.

Wolff, K., and Honigsmann, H. (1971) Permeability of the epidermis and the phagocytic activity of keratinocytes. Ultrastructural studies with thorotrast as a marker. J Ultrastruct Res 36:176–190.

Xu, Q., Izumi, K., Tobita, T., Nakanishi, Y., and Feinberg, S.E. (2009) Constitutive release of cytokines by human oral keratinocytes in an organotypic culture. J Oral Maxillofac Surg 67:1256–1264.

Yamaji, Y., Kubota, T., Sasaguri, K., Sato, S., Suzuki, Y., Kumada, H., and Umemoto, T. (1995) Inflammatory cytokine gene expression in human periodontal ligament fibroblasts stimulated with bacterial lipopolysaccharides. Infect Immun 63:3576–3581.

Yang, D., Chertov, O., Bykovskaia, S.N., Chen, Q., Buffo, M.J., Shogan, J., Anderson, M., Schroder, J.M., Wang, J.M., Howard, O.M., and Oppenheim, J.J. (1999) β-defensins: linking innate and adaptive immunity through dendritic and T cell CCR6. Science 286:525–528.

Yang, D., Biragyn, A., Hoover, D.M., Lubkowski, J., and Oppenheim, J.J. (2004) Multiple roles of antimicrobial defensins, cathelicidins, and eosinophil-derived neurotoxin in host defense. Annu Rev Immunol 22:181–215.

Zanetti, M. (2004) Cathelicidins, multifunctional peptides of the innate immunity. J Leukoc Biol 75:39–48.

# Homologies in structure and function among mucosae: oral, esophageal, and vaginal mucosa

The oral mucosa shares much in common in terms of structure and function with the esophagus and vagina. As in the oral cavity, the soft tissues of the esophagus and vagina are everywhere covered by a stratifying squamous epithelium which is normally non-keratinized, although in the vagina this may tend toward parakeratinization at the midpoint of the menstrual cycle (Nauth, 1993). The epithelium is supported by an elastic connective tissue lamina propria, and there is an encircling smooth muscle layer. This structure will be described in more detail below.

## 9.1 ESOPHAGUS

The esophagus extends from the upper esophageal sphincter, which delineates it from the oropharynx, to the lower

*Human Oral Mucosa: Development, Structure, and Function.* Edited by Christopher Squier and Kim A. Brogden.
© 2011 Christopher Squier and Kim A. Brogden. Published 2011 by John Wiley & Sons, Inc.

esophageal sphincter, representing the junction with the gastric mucosa (Gavaghan, 1999). The organization of the tissues reflects their function of transporting ingested food from the oral cavity to the stomach. The extensibility and motility of the mucosal lining is reflected in the presence of a non-keratinized mucosal surface resembling that of the oral lining mucosa. This is separated from the submucosa by a muscularis mucosa, consisting of a smooth muscle and elastic fiber layer, which may serve to reduce the excursion of the luminal lining mucosa as a result of the contractions of the external esophageal muscle, consisting of circular and transverse layers of striated or smooth muscle (Fig. 9.1).

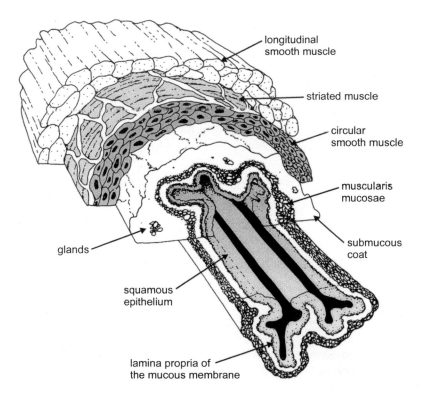

**Figure 9.1** Drawing to show the organization of the tissues of the human esophageal lining. (Modified from Gavaghan, Copyright 1999, with permission from Elsevier.)

## 9.2 VAGINA

The vagina extends from the vestibule (vaginal introitus) to the uterus where it surrounds the vaginal portion of the uterine cervix, a short distance from the external orifice of the uterus. The vagina consists of an internal mucous membrane with a lamina propria that contains numerous elastic fibers. These extend toward the external smooth muscle coat.

The mucous membrane is continuous above with that lining the uterus. Its inner surface presents two longitudinal ridges, one on its anterior and one on its posterior wall; from these ridges, numerous transverse ridges or rugae extend outward on either side. The epithelium covering the mucous membrane is a non-keratinized stratified squamous tissue. The submucous tissue is very loose and contains numerous large veins together with smooth muscular fibers derived from the muscular coat, which consists of two layers: an external longitudinal layer, which predominates, and an internal circular layer. The longitudinal fibers are continuous with the superficial muscular fibers of the uterus. External to the muscular coat is a layer of fibrous connective tissue representing the adventitia (Fig. 9.2).

## 9.3 ORGANIZATION OF THE TISSUES OF ESOPHAGUS AND VAGINA

As pointed out in the first chapter of this volume, the major difference between the mucosa of the oral cavity and esophagus and the rest of the gastrointestinal tract is in the organization of the epithelium, which reflects the different functions of these regions. The lining of the stomach and the small and large intestine consist of a simple epithelium composed of only a single layer of cells which facilitates absorption across the tissue. The esophagus and vagina are lined by a stratified epithelium (Fig. 9.3) composed of multiple layers of cells which show a non-keratinized pattern of differentiation, although this may tend toward parakeratinization in vagina during the midpoint of the menstrual cycle

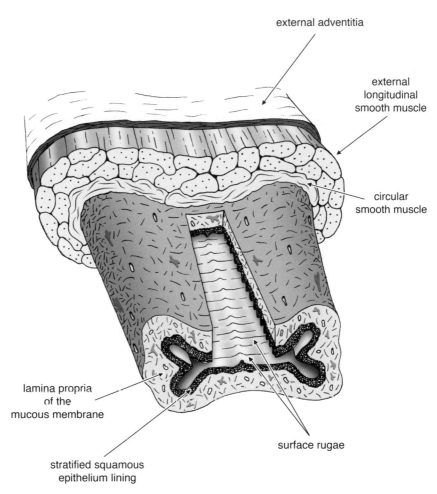

external adventitia

external longitudinal smooth muscle

circular smooth muscle

lamina propria of the mucous membrane

surface rugae

stratified squamous epithelium lining

**Figure 9.2**   Drawing to show the organization of the tissues of the human vagina. (Original drawing by Sean Kelley.)

(see below). The mucosal lamina propria consists of cells, blood vessels, neural elements, and fibers embedded in an amorphous ground substance. The lamina propria shows regional variation in the proportions of its constituent elements, particularly in the concentration and organization of the fibers.

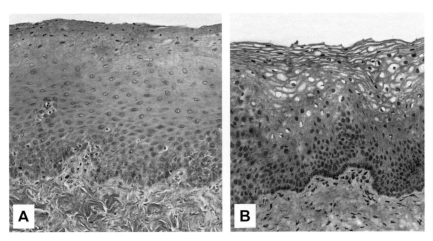

**Figure 9.3** Histological sections showing the structure of the non-keratinized mucosa of (A) esophagus and (B) vagina. Note the similarities with the oral lining mucosa (Fig. 3.1C).

The glandular component of oral and esophageal mucosa is represented primarily by the minor salivary glands. These are concentrated in the submucosa, and the secretions reach the mucosal surface via small ducts. In the esophagus, the minor salivary glands can produce a secretion with high bicarbonate concentration to neutralize refluxing stomach acid (Long and Orlando, 1999). The vagina contains no true glands and the surface moisture is derived from those in the cervix and uterus and from Bartholin's glands at the introitus.

In the esophagus and vagina, there are nodules of lymphoid tissue consisting of areas extensively infiltrated by lymphocytes and plasma cells. Because of their ability to mount immunologic reactions, such cells play an important role in combating infections.

## 9.3.1 Epithelial differentiation

Keratinocytes of the esophagus and vagina are capable of division so as to maintain a constant epithelial population as cells are shed from the surface. Tissue homeostasis requires differentiation and desquamation at the epithelial surface to be matched by cell division. Many factors, including aging and disease, can alter this balance so that an epithelium may become thicker (hyperplastic) or thinner (atrophic) than normal; in the vagina the fluctuations in estrogen production during the menstrual cycle also exert an effect on proliferation and differentiation of the epithelium (Schaller, 1990).

The progenitor cells are situated in the lower two to three cell layers; in the vagina the majority of proliferative activity take place in the suprabasal layer (Averette et al., 1970). Epithelial proliferation in the esophagus and vagina is controlled by the same biologically active substances, most of which are peptide growth factors collectively termed cytokines, as in the oral mucosa (see Chapter 3). Estimates of the rate of cell proliferation in various epithelia indicate that in general, the rate is higher for cells in thin non-keratinized regions such as floor of mouth than for thicker keratinized regions such as palate and skin (Thomson et al., 1999; see Table 9.1).

Apart from measurements of the number of cells in division (labeling index), it is also possible to estimate the turn-

**Table 9.1** Epithelial cell proliferation and turnover in selected tissues.

| Tissue region | Mean labeling index %[a] | Median turnover time (days)[b] |
|---|---|---|
| Small intestine | — | 4 |
| Floor of mouth | 12.3 | 20 |
| Buccal mucosa | 10.2 | 14 |
| Esophagus | — | 21[c] |
| Vagina: | | |
| —premenopause | 8.2 | 33 |
| —postmenopause | 6.2[d] | 27[d] |
| Hard palate | 7.2 | 24 |
| Skin | — | 27 |

[a]Bjarnason et al. (1999).
[b]Thomson et al. (1999).
[c]Squier et al. (1976).
[d]Averette et al. (1970).

over time; it can be seen that values for these parameters for the esophagus and vagina indicate a lower labeling index (and a slower turnover time) than for other non-keratinized human oral epithelia. However, because of the effect of estrogen during the menstrual cycle, cell proliferation increases in the vagina up to day 14 (midcycle and ovulation). This has been claimed to be associated with an increase in the number of desmosomes so that the epithelium becomes more cohesive and thickens from approximately 20 layers on day 10 to 45 on day 14 (Okada, 1990). Patton et al. (2000) have shown a significant decrease in number of layers between days 1–12 and days 19–24 although Ildgruben et al. (2003) were unable to detect any significant change in thickness between the follicular (days 1–14) and luteal phases (days 15–28). In terms of epithelial differentiation, there is an increase in glycogen within the cells and a tendency to parakeratinization. The reduction in estrogen levels at menopause results in a lower labeling index (see Table 9.1) and a thinner, atrophic mucosa (reviewed by Farage and Maibach, 2006). Thompson et al. (2001) have stated that the number of cell layers in postmenopausal vaginal epithelium ranges from 19 to 32.

Apart from the cyclical changes associated with menstruation, the principal patterns of differentiation are similar in the esophagus and vagina and resemble those of non-keratinized oral epithelium. During differentiation there is an accumulation of lipids and of cytokeratins in the keratinocytes, but this is less evident, and the change in morphology is far less marked than in keratinizing epithelia. The mature cells in the outer portion of non-keratinized epithelia become large and flat and possess a cross-linked protein envelope, but they retain nuclei and other organelles, and the cytokeratins do not aggregate to form bundles of filaments as seen in keratinizing epithelia. There are similarities in the types of cytokeratins in non-keratinized epithelia, but differences are evident between the esophagus and vagina (Table 9.2).

As cells reach the upper one-third to one-quarter of the epithelium, membrane-coating granules become evident at the superficial aspect of the cells and appear to fuse with the

**Table 9.2** Cytokeratins in non-keratinized mucosae.

| Tissue region | Cytokeratins |
| --- | --- |
| Non-keratinized oral epithelium | 4, 5, 14, 19 |
| Esophagus | 4, 13, 15, 19 |
| Vagina | 4, 5, 6, 13, 14, 15, 16, 19 |

Sources: Barret et al. (1998); Bosch et al. (1988); Moll et al. (1983); Tomakidi et al. (1998).

**Table 9.3** Permeability of non-keratinized mucosa to water.

| Tissue region | Flux (dpm/cm$^2$/min) $\pm$ SD for tritiated water |
| --- | --- |
| Hard palate (keratinized) | 1706 $\pm$ 93 |
| Buccal mucosa | 1963 $\pm$ 72 |
| Esophagus | 1220 $\pm$ 66 |
| Vagina | 4155 $\pm$ 70 |

Sources: Squier et al., 2008 and unpublished data.

plasma membrane so as to extrude their contents into the intercellular space. The membrane-coating granules found in non-keratinizing oral epithelia have already been described (Chapter 3); they have often been referred to as cored granules because of their appearance in transmission electron micrographs. Such granules have been observed in the esophagus (Hopwood et al., 1978), the vagina (Thompson et al., 2001), as well as the uterine cervix (Grubb et al., 1968). Only a small proportion of the granules in non-keratinized epithelium contain lamellae, which may be the source of short stacks of lamellar lipid scattered throughout the intercellular spaces in the outer portion of the epithelium (Wertz et al., 1993). It is the absence of organized lipid lamellae in the intercellular spaces that probably accounts for the greater permeability of these tissues non-keratinized tissues, although the least permeable of these do not differ greatly from the permeability of some regions of keratinized epithelium (Table 9.3), indicating the effectiveness of the barrier in non-keratinized mucosa.

The concept of epithelial homeostasis implies that cell production in the deeper layers will be balanced by loss of cells from the surface. The available evidence suggests a programmed breakdown of cell adhesion molecules, involving both lipids and proteins, probably by intercellular enzymes that might originate in the extruded membrane-coating granules (Madison et al., 1998). Regardless of the nature of the process, the rate at which cells leave the surface represents a defense mechanism by rapidly clearing the substrate to which many microorganisms adhere so that they are unable to produce toxic effects or invade.

# 9.4 NON-KERATINOCYTES IN ESOPHAGEAL AND VAGINAL MUCOSA

As already described in Chapter 3, non-keratinocytes represent a variety of different cell types, including pigment-producing cells (melanocytes), Langerhans cells, Merkel cells, and inflammatory cells such as lymphocytes.

Melanin is produced by the specialized pigment cells called melanocytes, which are situated in the basal layer of the epithelia. Cells with these characteristics have frequently been described in esophageal mucosa, as has melanin pigmentation and melanotic lesions (Chang and Deere, 2006; Yamazaki et al., 1991). Melanocytes, melanin pigmentation, and melanotic lesions are rarely observed in vaginal and cervical mucosa (Toncini and Innocenti, 1984).

Langerhans cells are another type of dendritic cell that are frequently present in the suprabasal layers of epidermis, oral, esophageal, vaginal, and cervical epithelium (Squier and Finkelstein, 1998; Terris and Potet, 1995). In vaginal and cervical epithelium, the numbers of Langerhans cells are highly variable, but this variation is not associated with stages of the menstrual cycle (Patton et al., 2000; Poppe et al., 1998).

The Merkel cell is situated in the basal layer of the oral and esophageal epithelium and epidermis (Harmese et al., 1999; Squier and Finkelstein, 1998). It has been observed in association with the rich innervation of the vagina after immunochemical staining (Hilliges et al., 1995). This arrangement is in accord with neurophysiological evidence suggesting that Merkel's cell is a sensory cell responding to touch.

## 9.5 INFLAMMATORY CELLS

When sections of epithelium taken from clinically normal areas of mucosa are examined microscopically, a number of inflammatory cells can often be seen between the keratinocytes. These cells are transient and the cell most frequently seen is the lymphocyte, although the presence of polymorphonuclear leukocytes is not uncommon. In vagina, there is a widening of the intercellular spaces after ovulation facilitating the migration of leukocytes from the lamina proporia (Okada, 1990). Lymphocytes present in vagina are predominantly CD4 or CD8 (Ildgruben et al., 2003) and, as for Langerhans cells, do not seem to vary in frequency during the stages of the menstrual cycle (Patton et al., 2000).

## REFERENCES

Averette, H.E., Weinstein, G.D., and Frost, P. (1970) Autoradiographic analysis of cell proliferation kinetics in human genital tissues. Am J Obstet Gynecol 108:8–17.

Barrett, A.W., Selvarajah, S., Franey, S., Wills, K.A., and Berkovitz, B.K.B. (1998) Interspecies variations in oral epithelial cytokeratin expression. J Anat 193:185–193.

Bjarnason, G.A., Jordan, R.C.K., and Sothern, R.B. (1999) Circadian variation in the expression of cell-cycle proteins in human oral epithelium. Am J Pathol 154:613–622.

Bosch, F.X., Leube, R.E., Achtstätter, T., Moll, R., and Franke, W.W. (1988) Expression of simple epithelial type cytokeratins in stratified epithelia as detected by immunolocalization and hybridization in situ. J Cell Biol 106:1635–1648.

Chang, F., and Deere, H. (2006) Esophageal melanocytosis morphologic features and review of the literature. Arch Pathol Lab Med 130:552–557.

Farage, M., and Maibach, H. (2006) Lifetime changes in the vulva and vagina. Arch Gynecol Obstet 273:195–202.

Gavaghan, M. (1999) Anatomy and physiology of the esophagus. AORN J 69(2):370–386.

Grubb, C., Hackemann, M., and Hill, K.R. (1968) Small granules and plasma membrane thickening in human cervical squamous epithelium. J Ultrastruct Res 22:458–468.

Harmese, J.L., Carey, F.A., Baird, A.R., Craig, S.R., Christie, K.N., Hopwood, D., and Lucocq, J. (1999) Merkel cells in the human oesophagus. J Pathol 189:176–179.

Hilliges, M., Falconer, C., Ekman-Ordeberg, G., and Johansson, O. (1995) Innervation of the human vaginal mucosa as revealed by PGP 9.5 immunohistochemistry. Acta Anat (Basel) 153:119–126.

Hopwood, D., Logan, K.R., and Bouchier, I.A.D. (1978) The electron microscopy of normal human oesophageal epithelium. Virchows Arch B Cell Pathol 26:345–358.

Ildgruben, A.K., Sjöberg, I.M., and Hammarström, M.L. (2003) Influence of hormonal contraceptives on the immune cells and thickness of human vaginal epithelium. Obstet Gynecol 102(3):571–582.

Long, J.D., and Orlando, R.C. (1999) Esophageal submucosal glands: structure and function. Am J Gastroenterol 94:2818–2824.

Madison, K.C., Sando, G.N., Howard, E.J., True, C.A., Gilbert, D., Swartzendruber, D.C., and Wertz, P.W. (1998) Lamellar granule biogenesis: a role for ceramide glucosyltranferase, lysosomal enzyme transport, and the Golgi. J Investig Dermatol Symp Proc 3:80–86.

Moll, R., Levy, R., Czernobilsky, B., Hohlweg-Majert, P., Dallenbach-Hellweg, G., and Franke, W.W. (1983) Cytokeratins of normal epithelia and some neoplasms of the female genital tract. Lab Invest 49:599–610.

Nauth, H. (1993) Anatomy and physiology of the vulva. In: Vulvovaginitis (P. Elsner and J. Marius, eds.) pp. 1–18. Marcel Dekker, New York.

Okada, H. (1990) Vaginal route of peptide and protein drug delivery. In: Peptide and Protein Drug Delivery (V.H.L. Lee, ed.) pp. 633–666. Marcel Dekker, New York.

Patton, D.L., Thwin, S.S., Meier, A., Hooton, T.M., Stapleton, A.E., and Eschenbach, D.A. (2000) Epithelial cell layer thickness and immune cell populations in the normal human vagina at different stages of the menstrual cycle. Am J Obstet Gynecol 183:967–973.

Poppe, W.A., Drijkoningen, M., Ide, P.S., Lauweryns, J.M., and Van Assche, F.A. (1998) Lymphocytes and dendritic cells in the normal uterine cervix. An immunohistochemical study. Eur J Obstet Gynecol Reprod Biol 81:277–282.

Schaller, G. (1990) Changes in keratin expression of human vaginal epithelium during different female generation phases. Polyclonal antibody studies. Gynecol Obstet Invest 29(4):278–281.

Squier, C.A., and Finkelstein, M.W. (1998) Oral mucosa. In: Oral Histology, Development, Structure and Function (A.R. Ten Cate, ed.) pp. 345–385. CV Mosby, St. Louis, MO.

Squier, C.A., Johnson, N.W., and Hopps, R.M. (1976) Human Oral Mucosa: Development, Structure and Function. Blackwell Scientific, Oxford, UK.

Squier, C.A., Mantz, M.J., Schlievert, P.M., and Davis, C.C. (2008) Porcine vagina ex vivo as a model for studying permeability and pathogenesis in mucosa. J Pharm Sci 97:9–21.

Terris, B., and Potet, F. (1995) Structure and role of Langerhans cells in the human oesophageal epithelium. Digestion 56(Suppl 1):9–14.

Thompson, I.O.C., van der Bijl, P., van Wyk, C.W., and van Eyk, A.D. (2001) A comparative light-microscopic, electron-microscopic and chemical study of human vaginal and buccal epithelium. Arch Oral Biol 46:1091–1098.

Thomson, P.J., Potten, C.S., and Appleton, D.R. (1999) Mapping dynamic epithelial cell proliferative activity within the oral cavity of man: a new insight into carcinogenesis? Br J Oral Maxillofac Surg 37:377–383.

Tomakidi, P., Breitkreutz, D., Fusenig, N.E., Zoller, J., Kohl, A., and Komposch, G. (1998) Establishment of oral mucosa phenotype in vitro in correlation to epithelial anchorage. Cell Tissue Res 292:355–366.

Toncini, C., and Innocenti, S. (1984) Two pigmented lesions of the female genital system. Blue nevus of the uterine endocervix and melanin pigmentation of the vagina. Eur J Gynaecol Oncol 5:76–84.

Wertz, P.W., Swartzendruber, D.C., and Squier, C.A. (1993) Regional variation in the structure and permeability of oral mucosa and skin. Adv Drug Del Rev 12:1–12.

Yamazaki, K., Ohmori, T., Kumagai, Y., Makuuchi, H., and Eyden, B. (1991) Ultrastructure of oesophageal melanocytosis. Virchows Arch A Pathol Anat Histopathol 418:515–522.

# Index

*Human Oral Mucosa: Development, Structure, and Function.* Edited by
Christopher Squier and Kim A. Brogden.
© 2011 Christopher Squier and Kim A. Brogden. Published 2011 by
John Wiley & Sons, Inc.